THE PRIMAL PRIMER

THE PRIMAL PRIMER

SURVIVE ANYTHING, SLAY ANXIETY, AND EXIT THE SYSTEM

LUKE WEINHAGEN

Core Human Competence LLC
Roseville, MN

Core Human Competence LLC
2864 Churchill St
Roseville, MN, 55113
www.lukeweinhagen.com
Send feedback to Luke@lukeweinhagen.com

Publisher's Cataloging-In-Publication Data

Names: Weinhagen, Luke, author.
Title: The primal primer : survive anything, slay anxiety, and exit the system / Luke Weinhagen.
Description: Roseville, MN : Core Human Competence LLC, [2022]
Identifiers: ISBN: 979-8-9867612-0-6 (hardcover) | 979-8-9867612-1-3 (soft-cover) | 979-8-9867612-2-0 (ebook) | 979-8-9867612-3-7 (audiobook)
Subjects: LCSH: Self-reliant living. | Survival. | Life skills. | Core competencies. | Autonomy
(Psychology) | Self-confidence. | Anxiety.
Classification: LCC: GF78 .W45 2022 | DDC: 640--dc23

Special discounts for bulk sales are available.
Please contact Luke@lukeweinhagen.com.

For Shelby, Duncan, Agatha, and Birgit.
May you someday find yourself in a world of competent adults.

Contents

Tell Me What You Think

Let other readers know what you thought of *The Primal Primer*. Please write an honest review for this book on your favorite online bookshop.

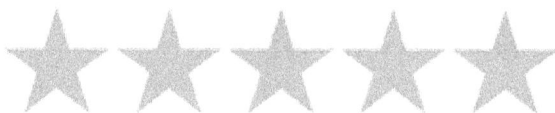

★★★★★

Get the *Primal Primer* on Video!

Luke Weinhagen's
Primal Primer on Video

Reading this book will not tell you everything you need to know. It will provide you with the absolute minimum core human competence. But to integrate this knowledge into your life, gain competence in these skills, and remember them when it counts, I recommend getting the videobook version of *The Primal Primer*. Reinforcing what you learn from this book with a visual medium—all chapters on video—will help *The Primal Primer* stick with you for life.

Thank you for reading this book and investing in your own core human competence. Talk to me anytime on Twitter @LukeWeinhagen or email me at luke@lukeweinhagen.com.

FOREWORD

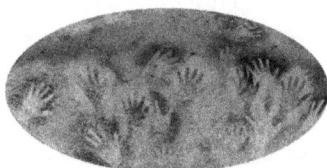

It is with great pleasure I offer the following foreword to this fine work: I am a family practice physician with a strong interest in complex systems, and how to improve them for the betterment of the individual and the community. It has been my interest, long before I went to medical school, to understand the complex relations between the human physique and emotionality. Along these lines, I encountered the work of Curt Doolittle, founder of The Natural Law Institute, in the fulfillment of the Natural Sciences with the proper incorporation of Human Nature into them, and so I began studying this in detail some two years ago.

In my efforts to understand and assist in the scientific works of The Natural Law Institute, and their publication of them, I met Luke Weinhagen, a man I identify as a "kindred spirit" of mine. I have studied his work in this common effort over the last year and a half, or so, and I have found him to be very interesting, in both his works and his character. He strikes me as the wise, stoic father-of-fathers type, who is quite quiet, then uttering a few profound words of wisdom that add great value to the conversation. His participation is always friendly, genial, and encouraging. In short, he is the kind of man that I would seek the company of, in order to refine my behaviors to match his excellent example, and I feel quite fortunate to share his Company.

In our mutual work, which is to operationally enact the Natural Law, I recognize the essential nature of what Luke is doing, as demonstrated by this book. Luke, a Marine veteran, has operated a Crossfit training establishment, understands just what it takes to physically train a human being, and has used this knowledge and skill to train people to improve their physical function. His skill set is wide, including the psychological, as well as the physical, in addition the entrepreneurial and social.

It is with this basic comprehension in mind that Luke has written this book, which is designed to expose the reader to the basic set of concepts and operations necessary to develop an intrinsic sense of security and psychological fitness for dealing with this complex and confusing world we live in. This book includes illustrative stories that bring what might otherwise be abstract psychological principles into the realm of the real, personal and tangible. This book will encourage the development of the strength of character and skill sets that will stiffen the spines of the independent individuals necessary for the construction of the strong society and civilization we desire, from whatever chaos might ensue from the critical times that we currently endure.

Enjoy the read!

—Bradley H. Werrell, DO

CHAPTER 1

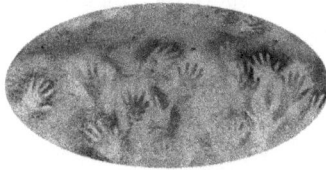

HOW WE FAILED YOU

Do you feel like society failed to prepare you for the real world? Do you have a sense that everyone else learned the big lessons, but they left you behind?

Does it seem like you're expected to already have everything figured out?

You've heard words used to describe these thoughts and feelings. Words like *anxiety. Depression. Fear. Self-doubt. Insecurity. Traumas. Triggers.* Some people you know even wear these as badges.

That doesn't feel right to you because you want to face the real world with confidence. You want to know that even if you don't have it all figured out yet, you are capable of figuring it out on your own. That even if parents and teachers let you down, you can lift yourself up.

You've already tried to take your future into your own hands. You took classes, went to therapy, bought self-help books, maybe even hired a life coach. You picked up a few tips and tricks to help you manage your "anxiety." That's the best they did, though, wasn't it? Manage. Get by. Survive one more day. Not alleviate, relieve, or resolve your anxiety forever.

Because they can't. Only you can. Here's how I know.

I became a father when I was seventeen years old. My girlfriend was sixteen. We became adults before we were adults. Talk about anxiety, right? In high school, I wanted to become a psychologist. Life had other plans for me.

My road hadn't been an easy one even before the unplanned pregnancy. I had recently grown out of the Dungeons & Dragons phase from junior high. (My girlfriend's dad was a cocreator.) Like most teenagers, I had no idea what to do with my life. I knew I liked sports and my girlfriend. But I wasn't exactly feeling ready or excited about being an adult, much less a father. And I was still dealing daily with the inner turmoil I felt over what happened when I was sixteen.

That's when my best friend killed himself. He left a note—it was all issues that feel important when you're in high school but feel like they're behind you the day after graduation. Like a hard breakup with his girlfriend, not knowing what to do with himself, and being frightened of the responsibilities of growing up. Some of the fears I had. His solution was permanent—solve the problem by never having to go through it.

To help us deal with the trauma of our best buddy committing suicide, the school counselor prescribed antidepressants to many of my friends to shut off their feelings. This approach sickened me. *How dare you diminish the importance of my friend. How dare you take my mourning from me.* If that was the official psychology approach to the problem, I didn't want to do psychology anymore. I became angry and disappointed in the adults around me. I disconnected instead. I took a turn for the worse. I partied. And I became irresponsible. Then my first child was born. I had no idea what to do. I did not reach adulthood with any better idea of how to be an adult than you.

I thought the best way to provide for a family was to join the military. I signed up with the marines right out of high school and served my time. A year after I got out, my girlfriend and I got married. We moved to Florida, where I got a chance to go to school and study game theory and game design. Gaming is just incentive engines with databases attached to keep track of progress. It appealed to my curiosity about human nature. And I studied programming and software development. We stayed in Florida for work. Then our second child was born. We moved to Minnesota to be near family, and I went to work. Years later, we had a third and a fourth. The oldest and youngest of our kids are twenty-five years apart. So at one time, we had an adult, a teenager, a child, and an infant—it felt like my wife and I were parenting four generations.

Throughout those years, I, like a lot of parents, tried to find a fitness regime I could stick with as a working father. I found CrossFit, and there I learned about general physical preparedness. Being prepared for the unknown and the unknowable—that was the early years before the games and the focus shifted to the sport of fitness. I got into it and opened my own gym. I noticed how people who stuck with it and got strong in the gym acted more confident, negotiated better, and improved their inner selves. They developed confidence because of their boosted physical capacity. I saw there how physical changes could affect anxiety, self-doubt, and trauma.

That led me to wonder what other skill sets besides physical fitness could improve a person's outlook. What about other confrontations? Other triggers we encounter? I began searching for ways to address those and found situational awareness (SA). That's all about walking around an environment where you don't know what's going to happen and being observant and prepared to act. To manage the unknown dangers in our world, we develop competence in SA.

I have adopted a term from my situational awareness training: "left of bang." We read text from left to right. Words are placed in sequential order from left to right. Disruptive events and occurrences that we cannot stop from happening are what we call the "bang." Our reactions to those events are on the right side—the wrong side, after the event happens. That's "right of bang." SA helps you keep yourself as far "left of bang" as possible. To prepare and act before the event.

For example, say a driver kills people in the crowd at a Wisconsin parade. If you had been on the ground, you would have heard a shift down the road from happy cheers to cries and shouts of dread. That's the first sign. Then the press of people moved away from the danger. You could see and feel the movement of the crowd. These are anomalies. If you're aware of the situation, you grab the loved ones around you and get back from the road immediately. You don't even stop, look, or turn around. You grab your family and flee. And you read about what happened in the news tomorrow after you've secured your family. You respond to the anomaly first before you get curious about the source of the anomaly.

People died in that Wisconsin parade, including little children. Those children didn't demonstrate SA because they were kids. Their parents also didn't demonstrate SA. Footage of the event shows people stopping and looking, not acting on the disruption in the environment. If anyone had heard the cries, grabbed their kids, and ran away, at least one of those kids could have survived.

That's what I mean by left of bang—act before the event rolls over you, not after it's too late. Pay better attention to your environment. Our brains want to dismiss the anomalies or get curious and stare at them. SA teaches you to notice anomalies and act before it's too late.

Once you develop SA, it puts you in a position of control over your environment and out of a position of dependence on it. Safety is in Abraham Maslow's hierarchy of needs. Remember that pyramid from high school or college? Basic animal needs are at the bottom—food, shelter, water. The second level is safety, protection, and security. Nowadays, people are dependent on their environment—parents, teachers, police, friends, a partner, an employer, et cetera—for their needs.

Dependence is unacceptable. The world will not keep you safe. You need to be in control of your environment. When you feel in charge of what happens to you, you feel cool, confident, calm, and collected. And when you feel that way, any feelings of anxiety, stress, or depression are reduced. It's not about reducing fear; it's eliminating panic to act with preparation and good decisions.

So how exactly do you relieve anxiety and other mental and emotional troubles for good? Just learn SA? That's part of it. But through everything I have gone through as a father, CrossFit trainer, and SA instructor, I have learned a harsh lesson: People have anxiety to the extent they feel incapable of taking care of themselves. It's all about meeting their basic needs—basic as in the first two levels of the hierarchy of needs.

Level 1: Physiological needs, such as food, water, homeostasis ("OK-ness"), and other basic biological needs animals have.

Level 2: Safety needs, including keeping yourself and your environment and property safe from harm and threats. This also expands into interpersonal relationships and protecting yourself from threatening or manipulative people, including how to persuade, influence, and negotiate with others.

The fact is, we as a society are not teaching these things. We don't prepare our new generations to live in a safe or smart manner. We're sending children into the middle of the road, danger is coming, and no one is there to save them. Not only is society failing to teach you how to meet your own physiological and safety needs, but in many ways, it's also failing to meet them for you.

Hence your anxiety. Uncertainty. Insecurity. Which is not your fault. It's normal. Rational. You're not broken for feeling anxious. You're in the middle of the road, and there might be a car behind you. You *should* feel anxious. You're responding to feeling blind and helpless.

At the time of this writing, my kids are twenty-eight, eighteen, five, and three years old. I have a twenty-five-year time span between my oldest and youngest, so I have a unique vantage point. And I'm forty-five years old myself. I understand what all generations under forty-five are experiencing and how it leaves us feeling naked and afraid.

Wherever you're at, I understand. And I know why you're afraid.

What's Missing?

Our society is expanding childhood into adulthood. We are undermining the development of the self—the responsible, independent adult self—in five key ways.

Dependence and Ostracism

In modern life, you lack the basic competence to sustain and protect your own life. You are instead dependent on others of your group for those basics, even others you hate. Ostracism from that group becomes an overwhelming threat. In our dysfunctional, dependent society, the satisfaction of needs requires you to constantly be aware of whether or not those you depend on for getting your needs met are amenable to continuing to meet those needs.

This is why approval signaling is prevalent enough to be called "normal" today. Everyone craves approval because they're afraid they'll die if they get rejected.

Reliance versus Dependence

Reliance on each other can start out largely well intentioned. Meeting needs is a good thing, right? But too much "help" has many of us living, acting, and believing like children. Not capable of meeting even our own basic physiological needs. Addicted to the subsidy and dependent on the providers.

At what point does helping become enabling? We'll discuss this in later chapters.

Boredom, Apathy, and Childishness

Childhood is being extended indefinitely into what ought to be adulthood. Imagination play is being validated like it is reality. Tantrums are rewarded with attention. All this results in a population increasingly incapable of independence.

One of the signals of this extension of childhood is when those in positions of authority, who appear to be adults but never learned to self-regulate like adults, throw tantrums. Pay attention to politics for a day or two and see how many tantrums you see. And these are from people ostensibly acting on our behalf.

Pathological neoteny is the term for this extension of childhood's behavioral flexibility beyond neurological maturity. We see evidence of the fanciful trappings of childhood replacing the responsibilities of adulthood where absurdity replaces reality. We now have adult humans claiming they identify as a half-elf demon fairy in a puppy costume, and they expect the rest of us adults to play along with their fantasy in front of our children.

Immaturity and Lack of Development

The immature (children) do not understand their dependence. The undeveloped do not take responsibility for their independence.

Immature and undeveloped adults mistake their dependence for entitlement. They refuse the costs of maturation and development and instead project them on others. That makes their problem into everyone else's problem. And society is sick to death because of it.

The Beholden Dependent

Someone in a state of dependence is not a person in control of themselves. They are not capable of self-determination. This person is beholden to their suppliers for the satisfaction of their needs, subject to the wishes, the whims, and the rules of those sources. They must forever appease the suppliers of their needs. This dependent person must prioritize their provider, be "other focused," acutely aware of others' attention, approval, and affection. Sacrificing their own preferences, ideals, and values instead of asserting themself onto their environment.

A dependent person is unstable, forever at risk of being triggered by environmental feedback. They live in a state of being perpetually afraid of the very society they depend on as it could at any time fail or reject them. They dismiss self-knowledge for external attention. They can at any time be completely disrupted by changes in their environment. The dependent person "needs" others; they never "want" others. The dependent person uses others as "needs dealers," as sources of supply. Relationships are about utility for satisfying needs, not engaging with others as nuanced and unique individuals. For the dependent person, what does not address a need becomes boring, irritating, or even frightening.

For the dependent person, those gratifying their needs are interchangeable. One adoration supplier is as good as another. Same for any love supplier. Same for any safety supplier. Distinctions become superficial. As long as the need is being met, who is doing the meeting matters little.

All this is killing our society and killing us as individuals. It's why we have the drug epidemic, overdose epidemic, and suicide epidemic. It's why we prioritize attention over connection. I wrote this book to teach you what I teach my own children. We will restore a core set of competencies that nobody taught you.

Wait, What?

You might be wondering what I'm talking about when I discuss basic physiological and safety needs. I'm not talking about toothbrushing, putting on your clothes, locking your door at night, or other things you learned by age four or five. I'm talking about *adulting*: that word we've invented for skills you should have learned long before adulthood that will sustain you throughout your life.

What differentiates us from other animals? Tools, language, and our ability to universalize what it means to be human. All these are things we learn, not traits we are born with.

There are additional skills we can acquire to make us fully developed humans—skills that enable us to satisfy our basic needs independent of external approval. These are core human competencies that were passed down for a million years. Only since the Great Depression and World War II have these not been passed down. Prior to that, people did not experience a world without that skill set given to them by their parents, grandparents, schoolteachers, and others. Depression and war left those generations unable to pass those skills down, disrupting a line of knowledge going back to the earliest humans. Baby boomers were the first to not pass down those skills. Now the line has been broken.

Look at the YouTube channel Dad, How Do I? as an example of people looking for means of learning those skills. Skillshare and other online platforms. YouTube tutorials teaching men how to tie a tie. The popularity of recent books like *The Subtle Art of Not Giving a F*ck* and *Atomic Habits*—all demonstrations of the masses seeking fundamental skills. Even Jordan B. Peterson teaching you to clean your room. Millions of books sold about basic physiological needs!

And then it got worse. The COVID-19 pandemic revealed the extent of the lack of basic skills when, for example, grocery stores ran out of toilet paper. And when produce and fresh meat increased in price by 25 or even 75 percent. People wondered, "How will I survive? How will I feed my kids?"

You don't know what you don't know. But part of you *does* know what you don't know. When you don't know how to meet your own most basic needs, your brain knows you're vulnerable. And that makes you scared. Anxious. Depressed.

So you've got to learn what you've missed. What generations before failed to teach you. As a result of learning these skills, even if you never have to use them, you won't feel anxious, depressed, triggered, aimless, or angry anymore. You won't fear the withdrawal of those things by others because you can satisfy your needs yourself.

What Kind of Book Is This?

This is not a survivalist or prepper book. The goal isn't to prepare you to go live in the wilderness tomorrow. But you do need to have the skills required in case you ever need to survive. Just knowing you *could* is the goal.

Self-reliance will release your anxiety. That will relieve your anger and release stress. It will do that and more by leading you toward independence.

So why this book and not just a YouTube tutorials channel? Those already exist. And you haven't watched them. I'm here to teach you *why* you should pursue those things and how they'll change your life for the better. This book makes those even more valuable and positions their work not as optional tutorials but, in many cases, as essential skills you feel motivated to learn.

This book will inspire you to set yourself free. And it will do so by teaching you the core human competencies that thousands of generations from the first Homo sapiens taught the next generation until World War II. Civilization drove technology, and technology required specializations. We overcompensated into specializations without a foundation. Now people don't think we could ever have been to the moon. We don't think the average man could have had a chiseled figure and six-pack abs without ever going to the gym. The bar is so low. We recognize the benefits of physiological health and meeting those needs, but we don't pursue them in everyday life.

So if this isn't a survivalist prepper guide, what exactly *is* in this book?

I mentioned Maslow's hierarchy of needs a few pages back and how being able to meet those needs independently results in mental and emotional freedom from anxiety, depression, insecurity, fear, and self-doubt. Broadly speaking, this requires the ability to survive. You need to know you can survive even if *everything* goes to hell, that you and yours will be OK. And it may get that bad someday. Civilization has marched right up to the gates of hell in the past couple of years. This is a new primer of the core human competencies that one generation taught the next for thousands of generations with such consistency that no primer was needed. WWII interrupted that knowledge chain.

Specifically, this book teaches you how-tos that were so important they were passed down from one generation to the next for every generation stretching so far back that the first time these lessons were taught, we wouldn't even recognize the species teaching them to its next generation as human. Go into any natural history museum, and you'll see the remains of these people—skulls and bone fragments and tools, marked with BC dates with so many zeroes in the year you have to do a double take in order to read the number. Deep time.

All the way up until eighty years ago. Three generations. That's about when we stopped passing these on. If we want to have any chance of surviving another eighty years as a civilization, we need these skills back.

If you want to live without a cloud of anxiety, the dread of uncertainty, and a sense that you're not sure what you're supposed to do in this life, you need this book. With these skills, your ancestors faced everything the universe threw at them. And by having them, you will feel like you, too, can face anything life throws at you—even if you never need to.

Because while you may never need to forage for wild plants to eat, hunt wild game, find a freshwater source, dig a sewage system in the earth, or survive the elements in the woods, the knowledge that you *could* makes you unstoppable. And when you feel unstoppable because you know you *are* unstoppable, you don't feel anxious. Or depressed. Or triggered.

And others will be comforted by your presence. You will draw healthy attention and positive regard from those who seek shelter and protection. You will be the person everyone looks to because you know what you're doing.

That is the result of what you're about to learn.

Why You Want to Know It (Even if You Don't Need To)

Why do we go to the gym even though our environment largely no longer requires physical strength? Because optimizing human physiological health requires incorporating these specific stresses.

Why do we need to be competent and dangerous even though our environment largely no longer requires self-reliance nor confronts us with perpetual danger? Because optimizing human psychological and emotional health requires incorporating these specific stresses.

Most of us recognize the former, institutionally down to individually. Most of us completely overlook the latter—and the dysfunction, anxiety, insecurity, and shallowness in our society tell the price we pay for this. To correct this, we must each become dangerously competent.

My goal with this book is not to advocate for complete independence by getting everyone traipsing through the woods and killing animals to get their own food, but rather to advocate for enough independence that if and when social disruption occurs, we do not end up in the streets killing each other for sustenance.

And I want future generations to have better mental health even if society doesn't collapse. Replacing helplessness and dread with competence and confidence will reverse our adoption of dependence strategies and restore strategies of self-determination. We'd end the extension of childhood into adulthood and withdraw the forbearance we ought to reserve for children from undeveloped adults.

If ending your dread and anxiety, boosting your confidence, gaining the esteem of your peers, and being safe no matter what disasters you face sound good to you, then read on. I'll show you how to become unstoppable.

CHAPTER 2

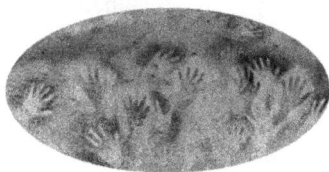

WHY YOU DON'T NEED TOILET PAPER

What is natural law?

The *Oxford English Dictionary* defines natural law as "a body of unchanging moral principles regarded as a basis for all human conduct." Which is a mouthful to say and a hard thing to conceptualize. We hear about immutable truths, but where do they come from? Nature? That's too vague. We need a clear definition to work from.

In its most basic sense, natural law is the application of the scientific method to the social sciences. We observe what happens between humans, test our ideas on why those interactions happened the way they did, and if those tests prove us right, we apply them as complicating factors and limitations we need to be mindful of to improve future human interactions.

Again, this is a mouthful. That's why I've shortened my definition of natural law to "the science of cooperation."

What does natural law, or the science of cooperation, *do*? Why is it important? What does natural law matter to you right now as you're sitting in a comfortable chair in a climate-controlled room and reading this from a tablet or a mass-printed paperback? What does nature have to do with you?

Everything. Because you cannot escape nature. You take your nature with you everywhere you go. Nature is with you as you interact with your loved ones and when you avoid someone you don't want to see. It affects your work life and your love life and your religious life. Someday, when our descendants explore the stars and colonize other planets, they will still carry human nature with them. That means we need to understand natural law so we can plan around it. We can never escape nature's dangerous feedback, but by understanding natural law, we can learn to navigate it safely.

I needed to learn natural law for myself because I'm smart, and I'm drawn to other smart people, but some of them are awful, and we don't get along. Why? Why are our interactions sometimes broken? I needed to understand so I could improve my connections with people and decrease the friction in my life and my relationships.

Over the last decade, I've studied at the Natural Law Institute. The institute is dedicated to discovering and sharing natural law and building social frameworks from a place of objective truth rather than subjective experience. Where the *Oxford English Dictionary* uses the standard "moral principles," the Natural Law Institute uses the standard "irreducible first principles" to remove even the subjectivity of morality. Their belief is "Truth was enough to create the West. And truth is enough to restore and preserve it."[1] Once I connected with them, I found a group of people who valued truth as much as I did. And I started writing for them by expanding on my concept of natural law as the science of cooperation.

Why do we need groups dedicated to preserving objective truth and natural law? Because some factors encourage people to reject natural law. These include evolutionary and epigenetic pressures creating truth that is uncomfortable to manage and also incentives like scoring political points,

---

1 - Curt Doolittle, "An Overview of Propertarianism for Serious Newbies" (blog), The Natural Law Institute, January 5, 2016, https://naturallawinstitute.com/2016/01/an-overview-of-propertarianism-for-serious-newbies/#gsc.tab=0.

gaining social power, or alleviating guilt by assigning natural status to unnatural choices. There are many reasons people might obscure the truth for both themselves and others. Though we may attempt to hide from it, we cannot escape nature's feedback.

As I investigated natural law and basic human behavior, one question haunted me: Why doesn't everyone develop agency? Agency is the ability of a person to look at any situation and say, "I can do something about this, so I will do something about this" and then act. Why don't all people grow into human beings confident they can control their environment and effect changes?

I said before that I disagree with some smart people. Here's the crux of my argument with so many thinkers out there and with other authors who write books similar to this one. Everyone assumes the bell curve is true, that people with low IQs already know what to do and people with high IQs can learn, but the vast majority of humans are in the middle and can never learn. Standard thinking in intelligence circles is that inherent traits are the limitation—that a person's IQ controls their ability to learn how to live better. Or that people are lazy and focused on the wrong incentives and cannot be turned. Either way, the assumption is that most humans on earth cannot be taught to develop agency and control their own needs.

I believe this is wrong. People can learn; it's just a matter of reaching them at the right time with the right information packaged in the right way. If we can approach people in a way that resonates with them, I believe anyone can learn agency. So I set out to identify what's getting in the way or what's missing.

That search took me years, and I can't recount it all here. But, long story short, here is what I found: people care when you make it personal. When you show them how they can protect themselves. And when you explain it in a way that gives them clear steps to follow, with no steps missed, so they don't feel overwhelmed. They take the instructions and the urgency to follow through, and they make it happen. And that provides the competence and confidence to make agency possible as they experience the changes in themselves.

That's what I'm going to do in this book. I will teach you why this is personal, how you can protect yourself, and every step necessary to achieve it. What you're about to read in the rest of this book is not just another to-do list. Don't think of it as "Oh great, more stuff to do today." Think of it as what every source, what every person you follow online, every influencer you like, every mentor you have, every authority figure you look up to and trust in your life has been telling you. Everyone tells you to do self-care. That's a big buzzword right now, right? Don't worry; this isn't about fuzzy feelings. There's a purpose here. Self-care in this context is going to keep your natural brain from destroying itself with fear. It's self-care in the same way building a permanent shelter puts your mind at ease.

This book is not a to-do list. It's a guide to primal self-care—the self-care approach that was passed down from one generation to the next for hundreds of thousands of years. It is the ultimate self-care list. That's beyond getting a massage or playing video games and drinking your favorite sugary soda. Beyond listening to a meaningful ASMR recording before you go to bed. Beyond going to bed before midnight. Beyond not being hard on yourself and all the other flimsy sorts of things people tell us to do for fuzzy self-care that doesn't really solve our problems. I call that fuzzy self-care because it's meant to give us fuzzy feelings, but it doesn't solve our true problems.

This book is not about fuzzy feelings. It's about primal self-care, which means tracing the methods our ancestors used to enact ancient self-care that kept them alive and at peace. This is Lindy self-care, Lindy being an adjective used to describe ideas and practices that work decade after decade, century after century, and keep coming up. They seem to find a way to survive century after century in a new society or on a new continent. Even if they disappear, they come back on their own because they're just so true. This is Lindy self-care. It's not going away, so you'd better learn it and make it work for you instead of working against you as it has in your past.

I don't want to tear down popular authors and influencers and gurus. But all those other self-care approaches are compensating for the fact that they're not solving for primal self-care. They're trying to make you feel better about the fact that you are not developing primal self-care. So much of what we do when we think we are taking care of ourselves is hiding the fact that we're not really taking care of ourselves.

Using my approach means curing the problem instead of covering it up with temporary fuzzy feelings. And that means I need to give you clear definitions, like I did with natural law. The same people who give you fuzzy self-care advice will talk about the necessity of mindfulness, but they don't define it. It's like meditating or yoga or something like that, right? Or listening to a self-hypnosis script or something? Or just not multitasking, not scrolling your phone while having dinner? They give us examples but not a definition.

And this was the starting point for my work when I looked for what was getting in the way and what was missing for most people. I inspected my kids' generations, because I have multiple children in multiple generations, and assessed where they were getting stuck. What was missing? And it was an endless list of fuzzy self-care that covered up the absence of primal self-care. Even if they did touch on primal self-care, they found no definitions to help them learn it in a context that mattered to them.

So let's talk about mindfulness. It's the parallel sister of self-care because it's crucial for self-care to take place. If I'm going to teach you primal self-care, I need to give you a definition of mindfulness.

Mindfulness is a clear focus on our present existence and driving goals without distraction. Regulation of negative emotion produces this state as it removes distractions like fear, which pull us from embracing the present to anticipating the future. Enough fear can cause us to abandon our goals in favor of temporary measures to resolve concerns. It is mindfulness that allows rational adult thought, the demonstration of ownership over one's incentives, which is what we call agency. We embrace the present, we focus on our goals, and we act on them with logic and reason in every circumstance. This is agency.

While each of us is more or less sensitive to stress, there are ways to manage our reactions. That's why I have intentionally sought out those skills I believe universally produce an emotional defense against stress in general and provide an emotional advantage in times of acute stress. A set of core human competencies that provide a foundation for the regulation of negative emotion, a necessary foundation for the development of individual agency. These skills are what I will share with you in this book.

To fully grasp what I'll teach you, you need other definitions first. Let's discuss maturity, independence, and cooperation so you understand how you need to prepare yourself to receive these skills.

Maturity

As individuals, we progress through a series of stages of maturity. Each carries its own challenges and features.

Infant

We are born into the complete stewardship of our parents. We hold no capability for self-determination. We can't even hold our bladder yet. Nor can we control how we act, which means we live with an external responsibility for actions where others are responsible for us. And we are dependent on our parents for both physiological and safety needs.

Toddler

Ages one to four continue into more complete stewardship by our parents. We gain the ability to act but still retain little self-determination. That means we hold minimal responsibility for our actions, and we are still wholly dependent for both physiological and safety needs.

Child

Ages five to eleven see us still under the complete stewardship of our parents. But now we are participants in self-determination and can even choose to disobey rules. That means a growing responsibility for our actions. However, a child is still dependent for physiological and safety needs.

Adolescent

Age twelve opens up a new world. We move from transitional steward-ship by our parents into limited individual freedom. That brings partial self-determination as we take control of some key choices in our lives, which, in turn, brings increasing responsibility for our actions. But we are still dependent on parents for physiological and safety needs, and if we make a mistake, we must remedy it with our parents. And we must ask permission. They still determine how much control we're allowed to have.

Young Adult

The late teen years should see limited stewardship by parents as the person moves toward full self-determination. We become individually responsible for our actions and must remedy things with those we wrong, moderated by our parents. We are now transitionally dependent on par-ents for physiological and safety needs but should be able to meet some of these concerns ourselves. We still ask permission for many things.

Adult

The shackles are off. There is no stewardship by parents, and we attain full self-determination. That means total individual responsibility for our actions and remedying problems we cause without any moderation. We ask no one for permission because it is our life to live or lose. And we are totally independent for our physiological and safety needs. Everything is up to us.

Development

As members of a social group, we humans have progressed through sim-ilar series of stages of social development.

Indentured Ward (Slave)

Early life in feudal systems was hard. Many people were involuntarily retained by their rulers, both centralized and local. These people had no self-determination and total external responsibility for their actions. They were forced to stay dependent for their physiological and safety needs and had no hope of redress.

Serf

Distance from their ruler granted a sliver of breathing space, but serfs were still involuntarily retained and possessed little self-determination. They were only minimally responsible for their actions, similar to a cat or dog. And they were still wholly dependent for their physiological and safety needs with no redress.

Indentured Servant

The ability to sell yourself into servitude (or at least the illusion of the ability since many couldn't survive without doing so) meant people were technically voluntarily retained. But for the duration of their work, they possessed little self-determination. However they were (mostly) treated as thinking adults and thus shared responsibility for their actions with the master they labored for. And during their indentured time, they were dependent for physiological and safety needs with limited redress for concerns.

Freeman

A freeman was exactly that: free. They even invented a word for people who attained separation from a master. It meant you were unretained and possessed full self-determination. That brought individual responsibility for your actions, with the trade that you were independently responsible for your own physiological and safety needs. And you finally gained capability for redress to the commons.

Citizen

The next step was to be unretained and possess full self-determination but also to be a deciding member of your community. That brought individual responsibility for your actions and your physiological and safety needs. It also brought pressure to insure responsibility for the needs of others via investment in commons. You had the chance for redress to the commons and could participate in political power.

Sovereign

Sovereignty is the adulthood of social development. You are unretained and can exercise total self-determination. That means you are individually responsible for your actions and your physiological and safety needs. You're also able to forbear someone else's responsibility. You insure the responsibility and needs of others via direct investment and can participate in the political guidance of your people. That means participation in rule, too. And you can redress grievances to the sovereigns.

The Cooperation Competence Stack

The progression through the stages of both maturity and development represents expanding layers of responsibility, the potential for reciprocity, and the capacity for cooperation.

I believe another progression exists, one I call the cooperation competence stack (CCS). This requires a person to do several things. First, they must become individually independent, which means learning the skills required to navigate the natural environment. This satisfies the first two basic needs levels of Maslow's hierarchy. Next, a person must become socially independent, which involves learning the skills required to navigate the social environment, such as managing finances, paying taxes, evaluating potential mates, and adopting norms. This stage satisfies the third level of Maslow's hierarchy. Third, a person must become individually valuable, which means learning the skills required to insure self-interests like identifying talents, learning how you learn, work ethic, and navigation of fulfillment. This establishes self-determination. Finally, a person must become socially valuable. That means learning the skills required to insure common interests like finding a career and cultivating investment into commons. It also opens up the secret fifth level: dangerous competency. This is proficiency across the three categories of human interaction—cooperation, boycott, violence—by developing the capacity to produce, contribute, and deliver reciprocity.

Our overdependence on the division of labor and overspecialization has us ignoring, neglecting, and dismissing the first three stages of development in the CCS. Those benefiting and profiting from our dependence prefer we skip the development of self-determination and instead focus entirely on becoming productive. Their model is for us to "go to school and learn only your productive skills, so we can tax and control you and your output." The dangerous competencies above are the elements the parasites don't want you to develop as they make you dangerous to them. Becoming dangerously competent requires you to develop self-determination. Self-determination requires a foundation of core human competence.

As I mentioned earlier, each of us is inherently more or less sensitive to the stresses in our environment. With competencies in place, traits like agreeableness or disagreeableness and other inherent characteristics matter less in self-determination. Without the stack, this trait matters more and limits dangerous competence to only the most disagreeable of us. It is this limit I am trying to remove with this book.

I used a couple of words you need definitions for: sovereignty and reciprocity.

In natural law, we define *sovereignty* as the condition of existential self-determination by self-determined means produced by reciprocal insurance of one another's self-determination by self-determined means, by sufficient numbers, with sufficient force, to guarantee it against those who would deprive you of it by the imposition of costs upon your demonstrated individual and potential group interests.

In natural law, we define *reciprocity* as the productive, fully informed, voluntary transfer of demonstrated interests, free of imposition of costs upon the demonstrated interests of others by externality and warranted within the limits of restitution.

Realizing all this made me search for a solution, which I found in Maslow's hierarchy of needs. What was missing in younger generations was not being able to meet their own basic needs, which prevented them from achieving self-determination. Why? Because certain key institutions benefit from your lack of competency. They revert you back to serfdom or social childhood and strip your power to resist.

The solution is to become dangerously competent to anything undermining you by developing core human competence. This means restoring basic life-sustaining skills that remove you from foundational dependency on external sources that want you vulnerable to manipulation to prevent you from fully engaging in cooperation. If you can stand on your own and join with other sovereign individuals, you can resist together what would otherwise threaten you.

I believe you can do it, even if you do not have the inherent traits everyone else claims you need. I believe you can learn the skills. I believe in you. I am going against my smart peers and betting on you.

Why do I believe? Because of Maslow's model of human incentives. Those needs drive our actions, including how we feel, act, and think about and respond to the world. If someone has a need and a clear solution they believe will satisfy it, they'll go for it. Contrast that with Freud, who believed through research on broken people that all actions are the response to trauma. That people are more inclined to give up than keep trying. Maslow built his hierarchy on high-functioning people as well as unhealthy humans.

Consider the hierarchy. It's a pyramid because you cannot meet the higher-level needs without meeting the lower-level needs first. For example, if you are starving and thirsty, you are looking for food and water, not thinking about self-expression and creating art. The model dates to a time when the typical person was capable of meeting their first two levels or were taught to by parents, teachers, elders, neighbors, and others in their system.

It's not enough to have your needs met. *You* must be able to meet those needs yourself. Otherwise, you feel like a slave to whoever is meeting your needs. That is where this book comes in. We need to free you from the dependence that keeps you feeling like a slave.

Dependance and Convenience

The typical person is not able to meet their first two levels of needs. We are dependent on modern conveniences. Consider the panic at grocery stores in the first COVID-19 lockdowns. People bought bottled water and toilet paper. Are you a functional animal on this planet if you are afraid you will be unable to use the bathroom? Dogs poop anywhere they feel like it and don't stress over it. In this way, if toilet paper shortages scare you to death, you have less sovereignty than a dog.

In the early twentieth century, modern technologies and consumer household products were called modern conveniences. They were not meant to be replacements that made us dependent on them. But we've become enslaved by convenience. We can no longer live without it.

Consider the first two levels of Maslow's needs: level 1, physiological, and level 2, safety.

Again, remember the bottled water and toilet paper rush in 2020. People were forced to recognize they don't have the skill set to acquire convenient water or convenient bathroom assistance for themselves. They don't have the competence to take care of their own basic animal needs. Your limbic system is aware you cannot provision your own source of clean water nor your own waste management. Most cannot conceive of how to provision those resources without the supermarket. Even *one* way of doing so would give you an alternative to the long supermarket lines and keep you resilient against shortages.

Where does your food come from? The same supermarket, restaurant, app, convenience store, or gas station. And people rage when they realize this. I posted in a Facebook group and said, "Growing your own food is printing your own money." Group members mobbed the post. Not only did they make it clear they are incapable of even a windowsill herb garden, they rejected wholesale the idea that the responsibility to feed themselves could ever be *their* responsibility. That means their brains were saying, "Not only am I incapable, I am not responsible for meeting my own level one needs. *Someone else takes care of me.*"

Remember this: entitlement, all entitlement, is based on an inability to take care of yourself.

We see the incapability to meet level 2 safety needs everywhere. Consider the current state of the first responder. No, I don't mean the cops or the ambulance crew. The victim is *always* the first responder. Whatever violation of safety occurred, the victim must respond. There is something you can do to respond to the event, to deescalate, to mitigate, to avoid. But the idea that the first responder is anyone *except* you is baked into our society. First responders are EMTs, police, or firemen. As opposed to you—the person threatened, attacked, injured, or hurt. The person who falls on the ice is the de facto first responder.

Listen: options of support are wonderful, but these do not take away your inherent responsibility. Consider solo survivor stories that go viral online—being your own first responder is so unusual, so remarkable, we have to tell everyone we know about such an event when we come across it. We love those "we delivered our own baby" stories. My wife and I did that with our third child because we didn't call the midwife in time. But we did it. Because we were capable enough to meet our own level 2 needs in that situation.

Most of us aren't. And our brains know this. So we live in silent terror.

The answer is to get smarter. Like our ancestors were forced to be. I saw a post on social media once that said, "Grandma survived the Great Depression because her supply chain was local, and she knew how to do stuff." That's exactly true. Your ancestors survived plagues and disasters and famine and war because they kept their sources local. Your great-great-great-grandfather didn't hear about a sickness and panic about how he was going to poop. He contacted his supply chain and made sure he got what he needed.

The more dependent on conveniences we are for daily life, the more dependent on conveniences we are to keep us alive. Prioritizing lowest-cost conveniences because they are necessities means that ultimately, these consumer products, the things we use and throw away because we can't think of an alternative to meet those needs that doesn't involve buying it from someone else, we end up offshoring our necessities (again, formerly conveniences) to countries that use slave labor. The current state of Western civilization is that we are dependent on slave labor.

Let me state that clearly: your life is dependent on slaves forced to work overseas for a global supply chain that can be disrupted at any time, either by accident or as a form of social control. We are so incapable that we're meeting our most basic needs with slaves and masters. It doesn't even matter who the supplier is; it matters who the cheapest and easiest to access is. Morality can't even factor in anymore. You get no say over your principles because slaves are keeping you alive.

To make matters worse, obesity, heart disease, metabolic health issues like diabetes, and all the other medical issues plaguing modern society show that even when we forsake the meeting of our own needs—our bodies' needs for vitamins, nutrients, minerals found in real, whole food—we settle for the convenient, low-cost, gross approximations. People choose artificially colored and flavored strawberry beverages over real organic strawberries. Growing up, my mom did in-home day care, and she had state nutritional guidelines to follow—ketchup passed as a vegetable. The institutions are not keeping you healthy because the healthier you become, the closer you are to reaching independence. Increased sickness means increased dependence.

Do you see the chains on your wrists yet?

The answer is to become your own master. To source your own solutions. Not to reject convenience but not to be enslaved by it. To do that, people need to be capable of cooperation with one another rather than dependence on one another.

It's not enough to have your needs met. You have to be able to meet your needs *yourself* because your needs aren't really being met right now, even at the lowest level. Our bottled water has carcinogens in it, ketchup is a vegetable, and you can't wipe your own butt if the teenager at the supermarket doesn't stock the shelf. These systems cannot support the most basic of needs, so they definitely won't provide you with life meaning—which is necessary for the higher levels of Maslow's hierarchy. Your own ability to meet those higher-level needs for yourself is dependent on your ability to meet those lower-level needs for yourself—or, more accurately, have the skills to be able to and turn "necessities" back into "conveniences."

You need to know you can do it even if you never need to. To end the lifelong fear that will haunt you until you learn independence and embrace mental adulthood.

In the chapters ahead, I will teach you how to fulfill your own level 1 and level 2 needs: your physiological needs for food, water, warmth, and rest and your safety needs of security and stability.

You can do this. You can become independent. And you can finally let your mind rest at ease with itself because you'll hold your own life in your hands without leaving it in someone else's care.

Let's start by discussing how you could survive if society ended tomorrow.

Even if it doesn't.

CHAPTER 3

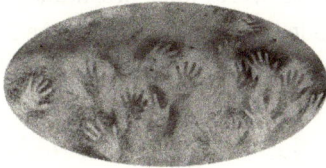

CORDAGE: THE MOST BASIC SURVIVAL TOOL

C ould you survive if the world ended? More importantly, what if you knew you could? What if everything went south, but you knew you could make it?

After this chapter, you will. Because you'll know how to make the most fundamental survival tool in human history—cordage. With cordage, you could build a house, drag heavy objects, or tie gear to your body.

Our ancestors knew this. The oldest piece of rope ever found was discovered in a cave in France. The ancient fibers had been twisted into what we call an S-twist by holding them together and turning them counterclockwise. Three S-twist cords had been twisted together in a clockwise motion, what we call a Z-twist. It's likely that homo sapiens didn't create this; Neanderthals did. Meaning that the rope-making techniques we still use today were invented by a species that predates humanity.[2]

---

2 - Michael Le Page, "Oldest Ever Piece of String Was Made by Neanderthals 50,000 Years Ago," NewScientist, April 9, 2020, https://www.newscientist.com/article/2240117-oldest-ever-piece-of-string-was-made-by-neanderthals-50000-years-ago/.

Think about that for a moment. Rope is so important that it predates our species. We've found even older impressions of rope left in stone dating back to 1.8 million years ago. Rope predates fire. Even some advanced primates can create makeshift cordage as rudimentary tools to help them get food. The concept of rope is built into our DNA. It's the second-oldest skill in the world after prostitution. And the first guy to make rope probably traded that rope to experience the world's oldest skill.

Can you make rope? Probably not. Most can't. You can't even create something so crucial to your survival that creatures with subhuman intelligence can make it. And your brain knows this.

In this chapter, we're going to fix that. I'm going to teach you the rope-making skill called cordage. Cordage describes fibers woven together that will not unravel. String, yarn, rope—everything premodern clothing was made of. Cordage matters because you can make shelter, make traps for animals, go fishing, weave fabrics, make clothing, hold up your pants, lace your shoes, suture a wound, sew fabrics or animal skins together, make baskets, and perform a thousand other tasks you don't even realize are based on cordage.

Consider what we use knives for: to separate things that nature meant to be attached. Cordage is the opposite—attaching things that nature did not intend to be attached. Cordage is how we create all the other tools. Ever see a sharp rock tied to a stick to make a spear and wonder where they got the rope to tie the spear together? That's basic cordage. It's how we corral nature, tame reality, and civilize the wild. Cordage enables you to meet the other needs. Cordage facilitates survival. It's the first convenience humankind created because it makes other tasks easier.

Once you master cordage, you'll have taken your first step to surviving no matter what happens to the world. And your brain will log the change.

How to Make Your Own Cord in Two Simple Steps

It's time to prove you're smarter than an ape. At least a Neanderthal. I'm going to give you two simple steps to follow that will help you make your own rope. You can do this while you're sitting in front of your favorite TV show or while listening to an audiobook. You can even use this skill as a fidget task in class or when you're bored. And by learning this skill, you can turn the ropes you make into cool items, maybe even bracelets for friends and family. There's nothing you can't accomplish with enough rope.

To start, you're going to collect materials. Then you're going to turn them into rope. As you collect materials, go in assuming you will make something six to eight inches long, like a lanyard or bookmark, and about as thick. It's OK if you collect more materials than you need because that just turns into more rope, which, in a survival situation, would mean easier survival.

Step 1: Acquire Materials

To make rope, you need resources. And if you're in a survival situation, that means using what's available in your natural world. So get yourself ready for a foraging adventure.

You've got a number of options. The strongest and easiest to find is tree bark because you just need to look around and spot a tree. Cedar is best, but pretty much any tree works. The goal here is not to kill the tree, by the way, so don't do what's called girdling, in which you strip the bark all around the trunk. Instead, cut off a branch and use that for material. The thin outer bark dries out fast and breaks like leaves, but the inner bark is more durable. Strip the weak outer bark to expose the dry inner bark, called the cambium. By scraping long strips of cambium with a knife, you acquire the material for making rope.

Another option is stalk fibers: things that aren't trees but grow leaves on them from stalks. Longer stalks are better for fibrous material, so taller plants are your best option. These stalks hold a cellulose casing that waterproofs the plants. Depending on how green they are, either crush, pound, or slice to open them up. Once you get them open, you'll see a pithy, woody, cork-like material. It snaps pretty easily. Snap the inner wood, then peel it off. Dogwood has been used for centuries, and scientists even found a 4,000-year-old dogwood net, so this stuff can last forever. The best stalk fibers leaf in pairs, and their seeds come in pods. They'll have cottony, dandelion-like seeds. Like yuca. It's a thicker fiber but could work. Again, the longer the better. That will make it stronger and more versatile.

If all else fails, you can even use grass fibers. Think wild grasses—the longer stuff, not your backyard lawn. Grass fibers can still be woven together into a strong rope, but it's the weakest option of the three. Go to the nearest meadow at a park, a Metropark, or hiking trails. Look for open spaces with tall grass up to your thigh.

When selecting your materials, avoid anything desiccated. That means dried out completely, which means it has been dead for years. Desiccated material falls apart too easily. You don't want your rope crumbling in your hands or snapping when you need it to hold. You also don't want your material too moist, fresh, or green. Good rope material is not too dry and not too wet.

Once you've gathered raw materials—inner bark, stalks, grasses—scrape off any outer casings with a knife, sharp stone, or even your fingernails. Neanderthals used chipped rocks as a knife for this purpose. You want the fibers clean, so get right down to the fibers themselves. If you find there's a lot of starch in the plant, then soak the fibers in water for a week or boil them for twenty minutes. You don't have to use a food pot for soaking. Old-timers just find a pond and stick them out there for a week. If you find cattails, you can simply remove the material and soak them right where they were growing. Or get a mixing bowl of water and do it at home.

You're going to start noticing raw materials for cordage everywhere. The fundamental building material of our species is all around you. You'll be sitting in class or walking out of work and say, "I could make rope out of that plant over there." That tells your brain you could survive anywhere.

Once you've stripped and soaked your materials as needed, you want to get them as dry as possible. A dead tree's inner bark will be dry already, but fresh plants will need time to dry. Place them somewhere dry—maybe roll out a towel on your windowsill so the sun gets to the materials—and leave them for a few days. It might even take a week if the material had to soak.

Once the fibers are dry, pick up a clump and rub and roll them back and forth with your fingers or palm. Imagine you're using a stick and some kindling to start a fire with friction or one of those propeller toys that take flight for a few seconds when you roll it between your hands quickly. The goal is to create friction. The friction buffs the fibers. What you're doing is getting all the remaining non-useful material off your fibers. Could be leftover bark, bits of inner wood, or some starch.

Now you have a bundle of dry, fibrous material—raw materials for cordage. You're ready to make rope.

But first let's talk about salvageable materials before we get to step 2. You can salvage plastic bags, old clothes, and worn and torn rope. Imagine a breakdown-of-the-world scenario. Pick your favorite—nuclear World War III, zombie apocalypse, or whatever social collapse is popular this year. Even in the worst case, you'd have tons of premade materials all around you. Those would break down over time, so you'd need to make repairs and turn old items into new useful tools.

Bags are everywhere in our society, and they'll probably outlive all of us, so no matter what happens, you'll probably be able to find one. You can also get hold of one right now with zero prep work. Here's how to break down a plastic bag for rope. Hold the bag upside down so the bottom seam is in front of you. Cut an inch off the bottom so it's a long plastic tube. Then cut long strips of that plastic so you've got thick plastic ribbons the width of your finger.

Here's the cool part—the length of your starting material will depend on how big the original bag is. Grocery bags are cool for small ropes when you need delicate tools while trash bags are better for more durable construction fibers. If you're building a shelter, use trash bag strips.

You can find them in any dumpster or trash heap, even at the end of the world. Making a small rope to replace thread? Grocery store bags might be delicate enough to sew with or maybe even use as suturing thread to close a wound.

Rope made from plastic bags is really no different from the nylon rope at the store. And you don't have to Bear Grylls your way into the dark and wild forest to find the raw materials from nature. Use what your world provides in abundance, which right now is used plastic.

Step 2: Attach Materials

There are a hundred ways to weave rope. And dozens of types of knots, some with awesome names. Whole books have been written on the subject of rope. I encourage you to spend some time on the internet and learn a bit about weaving and knots.

Today, I'm going to teach you a simple weaving method you can use to survive in any circumstance. It's called the two-braid weave. This weave creates a high-strength rope with low stretch. This applies to natural materials and those salvaged materials, so you can use it on anything you find. You can even do this with human hair to keep it out of your face.

To start, take a little bundle of material—maybe three to six fibers, depending on how thick you want your rope—and hold it in both hands. Put your hands at one-third and two-thirds of the length so you divide the whole bundle into thirds with your grip. Find that middle start point and get your hands on either side. Then, twist both hands clockwise—which means you'll be twisting your hands in opposite directions. Twist that material against itself. You're just twisting the material over and over and over until it forms a round cord instead of being a loose bundle.

Now, instead of just leaving the whole cord twisted, you're also going to fold the cord over on itself. After several good twists, you should have a segment of twisted cord a couple of inches long. Twist that into a loop and fold the cord on itself to make a ring at the end. This will bring the two long ends of the material together with the ring at one end, probably your left if you're right handed.

As you continue, twist only the top strand each time. Twist that top strand a few times first, then twist the two lengths of material together once in the opposite direction. Now the bottom strand is on top. Twist that one a few times, then twist the two strands once. The original top strand is now on top again. Twist one strand; twist the whole cord. Twist one strand; twist the whole cord. You're doing two braids at once, which is why it's called the two-braid weave. As you reach the end, you can leave it open or tie it off with a simple knot.

When you're finished, your cordage will look like a thick, round, twisted length of spiraling material. Just like a simple rope.

If you're a visual learner, check out step-by-step video tutorials online. Search "how to make wrapped cordage" or "how to make a two-braid weave rope" and watch what the person does with their hands. It really is just twisting the material, making a loop, then twisting one strand into the bundle, back and forth and so on and so forth. It sounds tricky to learn, but it becomes mind-numbingly simple fast. Do this for a few hours, and you'll be making rope in your sleep.

Note that if you're using materials that have *any* moisture, the rope will probably fall apart because the material will shrink as it dries, and the friction is gone. If you use green grass, it probably won't last a full twenty-four hours. You need to keep that friction within the cordage. That said, keeping a bowl of water nearby to keep your hands damp helps. A little moisture on your fingertips helps you more easily grip the raw materials without letting anything slip out.

Get this down, and you can do it anywhere. You can do this sitting around the campfire. Or twist rope and watch the river go by. Practice it while you're watching a movie at home. It doesn't take any mental processing once you've learned the basic movement. If you have two hands, you can do this. You could probably even use one hand and one foot if you lost an arm.

If Neanderthals could do it, so can you. Practice it now so you'll have this skill when you need it.

You Can Make Rope Even If You Never Need To

You may never need this skill. I doubt the world is going to end in a nuclear firestorm that reduces us all back to living in caves. The most likely time you'll ever use this skill is when you're camping, hiking, backpacking, on a fishing trip, at a hunting lodge, vacationing in a cabin, or hanging out with friends or family: anytime you're in the outdoors and there are people you want to impress, from your kids to a cute girl to coworkers or even potential clients on a work trip or industry retreat.

But you'll have this skill if you ever need it. That need doesn't necessitate the end of the world. Think about replacing a shoelace. If you're at work and break a shoelace, take a paper bag and recreate a shoelace to replace the broken one. Nobody carries extra shoelaces anywhere ever. Now you can get through a workday where you couldn't before.

And if you ever needed rope to survive, you have that skill now. Your brain knows it. The more you practice this, the calmer your brain will become. You'll see cordage material everywhere you go, and your steps will pick up a bit more swagger. Your brain will say, *See that plastic trash bag over there? I could use it to make a spear. If we all get bombed tomorrow, I'll go hunting to survive.*

And speaking of hunting, we'll discuss that later. We've got several other skills you need to learn first—the most basic survival abilities you'd need to even reach the ability to get your own food because you need to survive for several days before food becomes a problem.

We started with rope because it's a simple task you can do right now without too much labor or cost. Making rope is easy. And it proves to your brain that you are capable of becoming more resilient. By applying what you learned in this chapter, you've changed your own feeling of helplessness. It's no longer necessary to live at the mercy of your rulers or your environment. You've proved you can take steps to improve your own survival rate. Now it's a matter of how fast you want to learn the skills to become even more independent.

You've proved you can take the first step. Now you're ready for the more complex steps. Up next, let's talk about how you can avoid getting killed.

CHAPTER 4

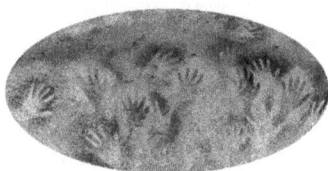

BASELINE VERSUS ANOMALY: HOW TO NOT GET MURDERED

The world works because the same things happen every day. We all behave in predictable ways.

Until we don't. And the world turns bad.

Remember the story of my friend who killed himself? I missed the anomalies in his baseline behavior. We *all* missed (or dismissed) the signs until it was too late. I mentioned him briefly before in this book, but there were pieces we missed. Pieces that can help you gain situational awareness in your own life.

This happened back in my high school days. My friend was a line cook at a fast-casual dining joint. Back then, real prep work was involved in food production, not just yanking bags from the freezer. My friend worked alone in the kitchen sometimes and had to prepare the food by chopping up meat and vegetables. One day he slipped with a big knife and cut himself so badly he received workman's compensation.

Except it wasn't an accident. He later shared with our close group of friends that he'd done it on purpose. He claimed it was for the compensation. But the workman's comp was only a tiny amount of money, and he came from a well-off family. The money shouldn't have meant anything to him.

This was the first anomaly. We all thought it was really weird, but what can you say when someone makes a bad decision? It's their life, right? Plus, he was a big talker. Always painting his every experience as bigger than life. It was easy to write off his admission as pure exaggeration.

Shortly after that incident, he asked around to see if any of us could get him a weapon. We felt uncomfortable about the request coming so soon after he hurt himself. He lied and said he wanted to customize it and see if he could get practice gunsmithing. It was his new hobby, he said. He went around to everyone he knew, friends and family and even some strangers, trying to find a spare firearm.

Second anomaly. But everyone denied the alarm bells or dismissed their concerns. His lies both times made enough sense. "This is what kids are into," we told ourselves. He was just being a teen, right? We all have weird phases. "He'll go back to normal soon."

He started saying he also wanted the gun so he could threaten the new guy dating his ex-girlfriend. We didn't believe that; we thought it was just chest thumping. He wasn't normally a possessive kind of guy. We figured he'd get over her, too. He just needed time. We shouldn't make too much of his claims.

Anomaly number three. And we still hesitated. Those three disturbances should have been anomalies we took action on. Our failure to act meant there was no opportunity for authorities to intervene.

He ended up buying a firearm illegally from a friend of a friend. His peer group was actually glad because it meant he'd stop asking. Maybe he'd calm down now that he'd gotten what he wanted. None of us believed he would ever use the weapon for anything. It was just more big talk.

A few weeks later, he shot himself with that weapon.

I'm telling you this sad story because people think situational awareness is about what to do in the event of a felonious assault or fatal weather event. How to handle problems when they come out of nowhere. But that's not all. There are slow-bang events as well. Anomalies can manifest months ahead of time, leading up to the bang occurrence. Remember left of bang versus right of bang? Everyone who does not act will say, "I knew something was wrong."

I want to teach you how to stop hesitating and start acting. When something feels off, you'll evaluate and act as necessary. So you can save a friend where I did not.

Baseline versus Anomaly

We always start with definitions so you understand exactly what I mean.

Let's begin with baseline. A baseline is what you expect to happen in an environment. Take a coffee shop as one baseline example. What do you expect to see happening? People sitting around. Machines whirring. Staff talking. All what you expect to happen in that environment. Your observations match what ought to happen there based on your experience.

Baselines are consistent anywhere. Coffee shops in Paris, France; Tokyo, Japan; and Raleigh, North Carolina all handle business the same way. You can walk in and expect to see orders taken, staff talking, machines working, and so on. Coffee shop stuff.

Next comes anomaly. An anomaly is anything that exists in the environment or in the behavior of people and things in the environment that either shouldn't be there or is missing. If you walk into the coffee shop and see an employee wearing a clown suit, you know that doesn't belong if it's not Halloween. This anomaly may or may not be a threat.

Context matters. Context is additional information that clarifies observed data. In this case, your brain sees the clown suit and starts searching for additional information that would make the clown make sense. What context could fit? Of course—it's Halloween. That context means you would update your baseline for what is normal at a coffee shop on Halloween. This is not a threat; it's just a seasonal costume.

Some changes are perfectly normal and don't indicate risk or threat. But taking one glance isn't enough. You must constantly develop new observations because environments constantly change.

Consider three example situations you've probably encountered.

Sirens. You expect a little stop-and-go traffic to and from home. An anomaly is sirens behind you. That's an anomaly. We have culturally adapted to that anomaly, meaning we pull off to the side so the emergency vehicle can drive through. Again, those sirens are an anomaly. But most of us just dismiss them.

Scams. A baseline on social media is to get a few notifications or a few new followers. But when there are anomalies, we often want them to be true. "This attractive person is messaging me with a great personal offer!" We want it to be true, so we pretend it's a good anomaly. No threat could possibly come from the hot lady asking us to send her money to help her get out of a jam. One of my family members fell for a Jamaican prince scam, not just once but on a regular basis, while he was in assisted living. We asked why he did it, and he said, "He needed help; it was the right thing to do." He got sick while sending them money and briefly went to the hospital, and the Jamaican scammers contacted local police to check on him. They didn't want to lose a lucrative mark. And he was completely unaware it was all a lie.

Sex. In the 1990s and early 2000s, roofies were common at sketchy bars and sleazy nightclubs. Special straws could identify if chemicals had been mixed into your drink. What's a girl to do? I tell my daughter to always drive separately from people so they are not dependent. You won't get driven out to the woods if you're driving your own car. Always check in with someone periodically—a girlfriend or parent. Doesn't matter who. Just check in. Tell them where you're leaving and where you're going. A white lie is OK—"I've got a work call to reply to." Keep dates where people congregate, especially early on.

The biggest tip I want to give you right now is that the worst threats pretend they're not an anomaly at all. They try to act like the baseline but think like the bad guy. They will want to win your trust fast and not break it too soon. And they will make themselves appear more vulnerable than is natural. They overshare. They may also lower your inhibitions by pushing drugs and alcohol on you. Basically, what does the online "pickup artistry" crowd teach about how to make conquests? Frequent but not creepy contact.

Consider a baseline for the date and for the itinerary. As one example, use a dog park for your date. Pick a daytime meetup with no rain. If it's getting late and it's rainy, those are anomalies to the baseline of the daytime dog park date. If he shows up without a dog, it's especially bad!

And that's a key thing to remember: people can say anything. But their actions give them away. Behavior doesn't match words? Bad situation. Like if you're going out with someone who says they're extremely religious, but then they try to have sex on the first date. Always trust their actions over their words. That tip is useful for *all* situations and with *all* people.

Situational Awareness in Practice

I can't give you exact recommendations for every situation you'll ever encounter because I can't define every perfect baseline in your world. So you'll need strategies to deal with anomalies. The following strategies, mindsets, and practices can help you make sense of your world and stay safe.

Restore Natural Curiosity

To map out your baselines, you need to be curious. Natural curiosity is supreme. Our minds want to fit things into patterns and dismiss changes. Natural curiosity overrides that tendency, so we engage instead of dismissing.

Foster curiosity to support being aware of your surroundings to keep yourself out of trouble. The more naturally curious you stay, the less likely you are to dismiss anomalies. Be "left of bang"—aware enough of your surroundings to keep yourself out of trouble. Don't dismiss any indication something is off. Pull on that thread to see if anything unravels.

In particular, obey the rule of three: if you hit three anomalies, you must take an action. Don't wait for three if fewer anomalies justify action, as in the case of one big anomaly. But don't let more than three accumulate before you take action. For most, one will be enough. But even if the first three seem innocent and nonthreatening, you still must act. It's never too early to keep yourself safe. You can always apologize later if you're wrong, but you can't bring yourself or your friend back to life.

I'll tell you another story. I knew a veteran who went on combat patrols in Iraq. Everybody in one particular village flipped them off or threw rocks at their vehicles. That was the baseline. Then one day, one guy in the crowd smiled and waved. That was the first time someone had been nice. They approached him, hoping he was friendly.

Sometimes it's a "good" thing that is the anomaly.

In this case, the friendly face was there to lure them in. There was an IED planted in the ground that they would have triggered before they reached the nice guy. The patrol felt something was off, so they stayed alert. That helped them spot the danger in time and narrowly avoid death.

Your gut instinct is a gift from your ancestors. We are creatures of habit. Intuition—the limbic system in the midbrain—is even older than our species. Our prefrontal cortex is effective at explaining away or denying what the gut says. Train your gut, then trust it. Curiosity will help you apply these gut feelings to the anomalies you notice.

Threat Decision Equations

Once you've got your baseline, fostered curiosity, and noticed an anomaly, follow this equation:

Baseline + Anomaly = Decision

The decision may be to get out as fast as possible if there's an observable threat equal to that reaction. But many times you'll want to gather more context. Why is that guy wearing a clown suit? What day is it?

Overreactions follow this equation:

Lack of Understanding + Fear = Exaggeration of the threat or dismissal of the threat

So get more information.

That does not mean fear is a mistake. Fear is often rational, and therefore, we do not want to compromise our fear response. But exaggeration and/or dismissal of anomalies reduces the efficacy of our decision equation. So in order to not exaggerate or dismiss, overreact or underreact, we have to adjust the understanding side of the equation.

Primal Situational Awareness

The situational awareness we are trying to develop when around people is the practice of real-time behavioral analysis because people behave in observable patterns. We are creatures of habit. Our behaviors are nonrandom. Our behaviors are difficult to unlearn and change. If we experience an internal change, our behavior changes.

The application of real-time behavioral analysis can be expressed as the "hunter mindset." (I prefer to call it the guardian mindset as my focus is self, not prey.) You may not feel like it today, but you have all the tools and equipment you need to be an apex predator. I don't mean this in the sense of you killing or taking advantage of weaker prey, but we evolved to be acutely aware of our environment and to notice even the smallest changes in it. This primal situational awareness provided us the context to anticipate and to predict where both threats and resources will be, thus moving us to the top of the food chain. All you are missing to recapture that ability is the skill.

With primal situational awareness:

- We think like the apex predator.
- We proactively search for anomalies and threats.
- We practice thinking like the bad guys (also called "red hat" practice).
- We do not dismiss anomalies so we can act on them like a predator, rather than reacting to them like prey.
- We bring environmental (contextual) adaptation to our observations.

That last piece is key. Everyone we observe has basic needs that must be met, like food, water, shelter. And more, too. We've discussed Maslow's hierarchy of needs. We use these needs to predict where resources and threats may come from. Because our limbic system is what drives our threat and survival responses, there are some hardwired behaviors and physiological changes consistent across all people.

When you see a change, go primal. Ask what the need is that has changed. What is the organism trying to accomplish with their change? What need are they fulfilling? This can help you avoid most scams and traps as long as you pay attention to actions instead of words.

Speeding Up Decision-Making

Situational awareness is ultimately a tool used to inform decision-making. We want to bring in observations about our surroundings and the people in them to allow us to make decisions as early as possible. Developing this skill is important not just in response to threats but also in taking advantage of opportunities.

There are five key steps to making faster and smarter decisions. First, proactively search for changes or anomalies in your environment, including in the behavior of the people in it. Second, apply your techniques of observation broadly instead of focusing on any specific element of the environment. That requires you to get off your damned phone—this makes you a perpetual target. Third, identify and evaluate anomalies fully to discern any threats. If you find no threat, only then dismiss irrelevant anomalies. Fourth, accumulate only enough cues to act. A 70 percent–informed decision taken in time is almost always better than a 100 percent–informed decision later, especially in threat evaluation. And finally, based on your observations, make a reasonable and adaptable inference. That means you decide what to do based on your data and then do it.

Act. That's the whole point of speeding up your decisions: to get to the action part in time. Nothing can save you if you don't act.

Deepening Context

You are not limited to your own experiences in developing your context. Each experience represents a file folder that informs your baseline for future similar experiences. In addition to your own file folders, you can add the experiences or file folders of others to add depth to the context that informs your baseline. Each of these adds to your ability to triangulate context when confronted with unfamiliar elements of new experiences.

It is like playing connect-the-dots as a child. Each folder you add represents another dot. And the more dots you collect, the clearer the picture becomes.

Take care to only incorporate file folders from trusted sources. Every folder is either good (direct personal experiences that were survived), bad (video games and movies), or incomplete (something trained for but not experienced). Curate your sources.

On Denial and Dismissal

You must train yourself to intentionally look around. And not just look but really observe. It takes practice to develop the skill to see what is going on in your environment.

Denial or dismissal is the first phase of decision-making. We reject most things as unimportant to what we're thinking about right now. This is automatic. This is also why "freeze" is the most basic of the "fight/flight/freeze" response. We struggle to process because we aren't in observation mode. Denial/dismissal is the most dangerous phase of decision-making as it can paralyze you from taking action, and delay can be deadly.

Denial/dismissal occurs every time we observe any nonstandard element or behavior in our environment. The "I just thought it was . . ." excuse after a threat situation turns into an event is the result of this denial/dismissal. To beat this, you need to practice not denying or dismissing. This goes back to curiosity, but it also requires you to actively engage with that curiosity. Lean into your observations. Look around you. Keep your head on a swivel.

A Situational Awareness Exercise

Go to your familiar restaurant, park, or coffee shop. Just pick whatever is easiest or somewhere you know what to expect. Get there and observe the present baseline. Write down your observations, and be as detailed as you can get: "There are two baristas behind the register making drinks. Machines are whirring every couple of minutes. Between four and eight people are usually standing in line. Half the tables are filled. Everyone looks relaxed and is talking or reading. No one is clustered by the door."

Then the next day, or whenever you can, go to a new and different place that is just like the one you visited. A different coffee shop, for example. Note any and every anomaly that's different from the baseline you observed in the first location. There may be none on the surface. But there are probably a few, even if it's just the arrangement of the tables or where people are standing.

While you're there, also note anything that changes. A loud crash as someone drops a glass. A huge lunch rush. A thief waving a gun as he holds the place up (hopefully not, but you never know). Write down the changes in your environment. Practice noticing them and logging them. Get curious about why they happened. Write down what caused the anomaly, too.

When it comes to threat detection, we have our baseline, anomalies, and context. Context can either change anomalies to fit the baseline—the clown suit on Halloween—or confirm a threat. We also have the concept of relevance, like the guy standing behind the counter in a clown suit, and it's July 17. If everything goes fine and he acts normal, this anomaly might pose no risk.

The Anomalies I Ignored That You Never Should

After I got out of the military, I moved to Florida with my wife and daughter. Florida has theme parks on every corner. Those crowds with guests from around the world show you myriad baselines with near-infinite numbers of potential baselines.

So there I was at a theme park for dinner with my wife and a friend who ran a martial arts studio. During our walk home after dinner, a group of guys heckled us. That was an anomaly. We ignored it. Just kept walking back to the parking lot. Walking took us farther away from people.

The guys kept following us. That was the *second* anomaly, which we also dismissed. "Oh, they're just going to the parking lot, too."

No. As it turned out, they were stalking us. The guys confronted us as soon as we got out of earshot and eyesight of the crowd. I tried to de-escalate the situation, but this was a bang event. I stepped in front of my wife to keep them away from her. Then one attacker threw a punch at my friend, who blocked it. I grabbed the other punk, threw him to the ground, and jumped on top of him. Meanwhile, my martial artist friend battled his attacker.

My military background and my martial artist friend's background were not the right fit for these jerks. We terrified them. They broke off and ran away.

After the event, my wife was shaken up. She'd been training in martial arts at the time, so she wasn't completely at an attacker's mercy, but she had never been in an altercation before. It takes time to calm down from an experience like that, and eventually, she did. But she knew it could have gone badly if we hadn't been prepared for the fight.

But what could have happened? We ignored verbal aggression and then ignored them following us. A bang situation—an attack—actually occurred. We could have confronted them while still in public areas and might have avoided the attack.

I don't want you to have to be in that situation. Respond to the first anomaly. All you have to do is circle back around to where people are. Even after the second anomaly, we could have easily gone back. We could have said, "I forgot something at the bar." The longer we let it go, the more obvious it was they were following us.

Returning to where people are reduces likelihood of an altercation because it raises the stakes for the attacker. So if you feel threatened, get somewhere where the baseline is stronger against changing, where you know you'll be safe.

This is situational awareness. And now that you know how to keep yourself safe, your brain won't need to be terrified of the outside world. You'll be able to figure out when you're safe, and I mean *really* safe, not just naive. Practice this skill, and your brain will learn when to relax.

CHAPTER 5

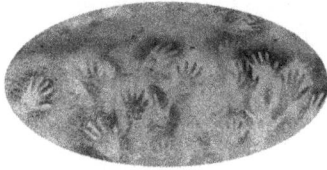

SHELTER: HOW TO SURVIVE IN THE WILD

It was New Year's Eve, 1993. I was sixteen years old. My girlfriend (now my wife) and I were getting ready to drive from Minnesota to Wisconsin. The sun had set. We could see our breath in the zero-degree air. I finished packing the car, buttoned up my denim jacket, and closed the trunk.

Most of my family lived in Minnesota, but a small branch had set up a hobby farm in the middle of nowhere, Wisconsin. Tonight they'd invited everyone to a New Year's party at their small patch of land.

My girlfriend's parents had let her join me on the condition that I bring her home the same night. I'd grudgingly agreed. There was no reason we couldn't have stayed the night. Everyone was sleeping in the same room, anyway. Nevertheless, I was glad to bring her along and show her how my family partied.

It was a ninety-minute drive, maybe a little longer with the limited visibility. No matter. I was eager for my girlfriend to meet my whole family. Maybe too eager since she kept telling me to watch my speed.

I'd never driven out there before, but I managed to keep pace with the other Weinhagens and arrive on time. It was great to have everyone together. And most important, it was a pleasure to introduce my girlfriend. She was a hit.

Before I knew it, the clock struck twelve. Everyone locked arms and sang "Auld Lang Syne." I had to get Cinderella home. Our carriage wouldn't turn into a pumpkin, but there was a definite chance of it turning into a popsicle. The temperature had dropped, and there had been significant snowfall during the party, too.

My girlfriend phoned her parents and asked if she could stay. "No chance," they said.

So I had to traverse the dark, icy roads. Piece of cake.

The cold air cut straight through our clothes as we trudged to the car with our shoulders hunched. We took off slowly and headed back to the Twin Cities. Driving snow swirled around the car, reducing my view to the twenty feet of road ahead.

I rounded a bend and hit a patch of ice. The car went into a spin, flew off the road, and crashed into a ditch. We wound up stuck.

This was the early nineties. Cell phones were luxury items back then. We had no means of getting in touch with anyone, and we were too far from the farm to walk back.

Throughout this book, you've read about being left of bang. Well, our New Year's was a clear example of what happens when you are not left of bang. Bad decisions had led to more bad decisions.

Here's where I went wrong:

- Leaving in the middle of a snowstorm
- Making the drive alone with my girlfriend
- Going to the party knowing we had to come home the same night

We should have put on a couple of extra layers or brought warmer clothing. We'd dressed for a party, not arctic exploration.

I had a choice to make: stay in the car and freeze to death or get out of the car, hoping to flag someone down. And still freeze to death.

So I got out, climbed up to the road, and looked for a car to wave down. When my fingers went numb, I returned to the car and warmed myself up. Then I got back out and hoped for headlights.

By sheer dumb luck, a bartender was coming off the late shift. Imagine leaving a long night at work surrounded by drunks, then having to help pull a dumb kid and his girlfriend out of a ditch.

Once the Good Samaritan had pulled us out, we got back on our way. Words can't express how grateful we felt.

It was pure chance that the driver had been there to save us. You might not be so lucky. Maybe no one comes, and your car runs out of gas. You might have your cell, but service is not omnipresent, and batteries drain fast in the cold.

Here's the takeaway: your survival from exposure depends on shelter. If we'd decided to leave the car and walk, we would be dead.

What Exactly Is Shelter?

Shelter is a simple word, but it can have different meanings. Some people say it's four walls and a roof. To others, it's anywhere that protects from bad weather.

And they're all right, but wrong in a technical sense. Shelters are not defined by their construction; they're places within which you can control the air mass.

Did you ever go on a school field trip to a cave system? Some have signs that say SIXTY-FIVE DEGREES EVERY DAY, ALL YEAR LONG. Do you remember how warm the air felt? That's because a cave is a natural shelter. And it's the most basic air mass management system.

What do I mean by air mass management?

Let's get a bit technical for a moment. Your body is hot, and when it transfers heat to the air molecules around it, the air heats up, too. This means when you put a jacket on, you're trapping the air inside.

That's why your mom told you to zip up your jacket when you went outside. It is not the jacket that keeps you warm; it's the air trapped inside.

In the same way, it's not the insulation that warms the house. It's the air trapped in the house by the insulation that keeps you warm.

It doesn't even matter what you use to build your shelter. Here's an example. I love playing in the snow with my kids. In Minnesota, we can get anywhere from thirty-six to seventy inches per year. One year, my eldest and I were building a snow fort. It got to about six feet high, with room for four people inside. Snow Fort Knox!

My son and I were working inside, carving out shelf space in the walls. Despite being in our T-shirts, we were sweating. My son was amazed that it was so warm inside, even though we were surrounded by snow. That's air mass control.

Knowing this principle may prove to be the difference between dying from exposure and surviving.

Environmental Threats, Practical Solutions

If you are caught out in the wilderness, you have one major concern. It's not wolves or even a band of marauders.

Your biggest concern is exposure.

The average body temperature is 98.6° F. The longer you're exposed to the cold, the more your body temperature will drop. When the ambient temperature falls to 50°, hypothermia kicks in. At 30°, you run a serious risk of frostbite. Any lower than that, and you will die.

The crucial step when dealing with exposure is learning what kind of threat your environment poses. If you're on the verge of being compromised because of exposure, you need to create an emergency shelter as soon as you can. This becomes your top priority because it will mean the difference between life and death.

There's no place for perfectionism when it comes to an emergency shelter. All that matters is that you get your shelter secure, then you secure yourself inside the shelter.

Emergency Shelter

An emergency shelter is the simplest type of shelter. It may be as simple as digging a hole in a snowbank like I should have done when stranded on New Year's. It may not seem like much, but a hole in the ground is a valid emergency shelter.

When digging an emergency shelter, use whatever you can: a hammer, sticks, even your hands. An emergency shelter's main purpose is getting you out of the wind because wind chill will make you feel even colder.

The same rule applies to high heat. Prolonged sun exposure can cause heat stroke or burns.

In a desert, it may be more difficult to find a suitable shelter. An ideal place would be a cave. If you can't find a cave, then you have to find shade. A rock formation that can keep you in the shade from head to foot may save your life.

No matter what, your main challenge is the wind. It is Mother Nature's go-to weapon in her crusade to kill you. The wind can articulate in various ways, whether as a blizzard or a sandstorm. It can carry particles like sand or snow, even branches that might concuss or, in extreme cases, impale you.

When looking for an emergency shelter, you must identify every risk and put an obstacle between you and those risks.

Temporary Shelter

If you are exhausted and are looking for a place to lie down, you need a temporary shelter. The point of an emergency shelter is to get you away from the immediate threat posed by the elements. A temporary shelter is a safe place where you'll sleep for the night.

You are at your most vulnerable when you're asleep, so your temporary shelter needs to be in a safe spot. Under a hornet's nest is not suitable; neither is the edge of a mosquito-filled swamp. People and animals can pose a threat to you, too. If either are present, you'll need to build something more inconspicuous, maybe even camouflaged.

Ideal Site Necessities

Let's say you're stranded but can pick a site for your temporary shelter. What would the ideal site look like? First, it must contain the material you need to construct the temporary shelter. If you have to walk miles to gather materials, it is not a good site. Burning up all your energy in procurement will leave you too exhausted to build the shelter. You'll also lose the daylight needed to build the shelter and spend the night exposed to the life-threatening elements.

The site for your temporary shelter must be large enough and flat enough for you to lie down and be comfortable. It's not going to be the Ritz, but it will help you survive.

You should steer clear of ridgelines and water lines. A ridgeline is the crest of a hill, cliff, or mountain. If you roll off the side of a mountain, your odds of survival will drop with you. Even if you stay on the mountain, your old adversary the wind will ruin your night.

At the same time, you don't want to stay in a valley basin because of the risk of flash floods. Stay above the watermarks. These appear as dark spots on trees. If you see hills or trees packed with snow, avoid sleeping right below them. All it takes is a little wind, and your body won't be found till after the thaw. Clues are everywhere. Always be mindful of your surroundings.

Contextual Requirements

Those were the hard requirements. The following are contextual requirements that layer on top of them.

Concealment. Does your shelter provide concealment from threats? Whether animals or other people, threats depend on the circumstances you find yourself in.

Exit strategy. What if you need to get out of the area fast? You'll need to plan your escape route.

Attention grabber. Is it suitable for signaling? Maybe you're not under threat from other people, but you need to attract other people's attention. In my New Year's situation, I wanted to be able to signal any kind of car passing by. The area you pick must provide you with the means of attracting the appropriate attention.

Protection. Does the area protect against wild animals, rocks, or dead trees that might fall? When you're scouting for a site, keep a lookout for fallen trees. They can only fall once, so use them as material for your shelter. You should avoid areas that are close to reptiles, insects, and poisonous plants, so learn about the flora and fauna of the area you will be traveling to. A little research may save your life.

Remember that animals need food, water, and warmth, too. Providing these necessities for yourself will attract most animals. If you have to leave your shelter for several hours, will you come back to find you have raccoon roommates? What about mice? When you leave the shelter, build the habit of removing materials. And always check for unwanted lodgers when you return. The shelter has to be warm for you and no one else.

Bedding. In your temporary shelter, you have to have bedding. Comfort is not the point. Trapping air to control the temperature is. Bedding also adds a buffer between you and the ground, which can suck heat away from you. Use whatever you can find to trap air beneath you: leaves, dried grass, even branches.

BLISS

To help you remember everything I've taught you so far, here's what I tell the students in my situational awareness courses: you want to achieve a state of BLISS.

What is BLISS? It's not euphoria; it's an acronym. I'll walk you through each letter.

Blend in with your surroundings. You don't want to draw any unnecessary attention to yourself. Survival depends on keeping a low profile.

Low silhouette. A low silhouette achieves two tasks. One, it makes your shelter harder to see. Two, it reduces your wind profile. That means less wind blowing through your shelter.

Irregular shape. Humans see patterns everywhere. If your shelter is asymmetrical, it is less likely to stand out and be noticed.

Small. The smaller your shelter, the easier it is to manage. A small space means less air you need to trap to keep warm.

Secluded location. The more out of the way you are, the less likely you'll be to attract unwanted visitors.

Frame Game

Now that you have a site, you have to build a temporary shelter—in particular, a debris shelter. Debris shelters are simple, sturdy, and versatile. There are two main types of debris shelter: the lean-to and its little brother, the A-frame.

Lean-To

Before you begin construction, ask yourself what direction the wind is blowing. The same applies to snowfall. The lean-to must be built between you and the wind or any other environmental concerns. Besides keeping you warm, it must shield you from the elements.

Once you know the location and direction for your lean-to, the next step is to acquire the raw materials to build the shelter.

First, you need a branch to be your crossbeam. A wrist-thick one is ideal. Make sure the branch is sturdy and not rotten so it can take the weight of the ribs. The crossbeam also needs to cover the length of your body so you will be completely covered. Once you have your crossbeam, look for trees that are close together. You need the crossbeam to fit between them. In particular, you want a Y-shaped crook in the trees so you can slide the crossbeam between them to create the structure's main spine.

Once you have the crossbeam in place, load up the ribs. These are long branches you set on the ground to lean against the beam: hence the term *lean-to*. Place them at an angle to block the wind and rain.

Now that you have the ribs in place, locate as many leafy branches as possible. Evergreen branches are excellent for this. Place the branches on the structure horizontally at first, then vertically. Once you have the area between the two trees covered, build another layer on top. Have at least five layers. Place them like shingles, and close over the gaps as much as possible so the wind cannot penetrate. Repeat until the branch layer is about a foot thick.

Layer the ground with leaves and branches. You've just built yourself a lean-to.

A-Frame

An A-frame is half a lean-to, with only one end of the crossbeam elevated. When you're building an A-frame, have the opening face away from the wind. If you're building in a desert or high-temperature environment, build it facing east to reduce sun exposure.

An A-frame looks like a single-person tent. You are applying the same principles as a lean-to, just half the size. The A-frame consists of your crossbeam and two branches that will form the entrance. They will need to be strong enough to support the structure's weight. Layer them up with branches and leaves as with the lean-to.

Which should you build, an A-frame or a lean-to? It all depends on what resources are close at hand. If you can find two trees close enough together to support a crossbeam, and if there is plenty of material, build a lean-to. If not, build an A-frame.

Remember: temporary shelters are for short-term survival before getting rescued or moving on to a new area.

Permanent Shelter

If you are going to be in the area for a longer period or if you are keeping or storing resources, you will need a permanent shelter.

Imagine you're in an emergency scenario. You dug your hole in the ground, weathered the storm, and now you have found a good spot and built a lean-to. As the sun sets, you realize that you are going to be here until the rescue party finds you.

During the day, you'll focus on making cordage. Use the cordage to lash your shelter's ribs to the crossbeam.

Wattle and daub is a millennium-old building technique that can turn your temporary shelter into a stronger, semipermanent structure. Wattle is a lattice wall made by weaving sticks together, and daub is a mixture of clay, mud, dung, and a binder such as straw or dried grass. The daub is used to fill gaps in the wattle like plaster.

A semipermanent shelter will give you the time to build a long-term structure like a wooden cabin. However, you would need a group to tackle an undertaking like a cabin.

Why would you need to build these structures?

Put it like this: if worse comes to worst, you need to survive long enough to find other people. You now also bring value to the people you meet up with. Being able to build semipermanent structures is a tradable skill. The war chief might give you a stay of execution if you can build him a sweet pad. Heck, you could be the war chief because you have the best shelter.

These skills are invaluable if you get separated while on vacation or backpacking.

The most important reason you need this skill is for your own peace of mind. If your limbic system knows you can survive, that is half the battle. Besides, it's good to know that when nature throws a punch, you can hit right back.

To quote my favorite poet Piet Hein, "Problems worthy of attack prove their worth by hitting back."

CHAPTER 6

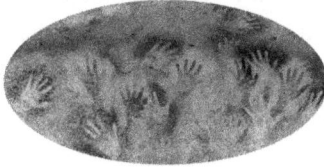

DISRUPTED ENVIRONMENT: HOW TO READ A ROOM

W hen I was in the service, I met a lot of different people and made many friends I wouldn't have otherwise. For example, I made good friends with a guy who lived close to where we were stationed in North Carolina. A childhood friend of his, a nice African American guy, invited him to a party one weekend. He asked me to come with him.

We made the hour-and-a-half drive and hooked up with his friend. The three of us started driving down all these back roads, which turned into dirt roads, getting farther and farther from civilization.

Finally, we came to a building. Maybe it was an old barn; I couldn't tell because it was dark. But we could hear music coming from inside.

We pulled up to the backwoods barn party and got out of the car. The driver, my friend's buddy, said, "Go ahead. I'll catch up."

My friend and I walked in. Everyone stopped talking, turned, and looked at us because we were the only two white people in the whole place.

After what felt like forever, my friend's buddy joined us. He introduced us, and everything went back to normal.

It was the most surreal atmospheric shift I have ever experienced. The mood switched from one extreme to the other because we entered the room.

Notice that the addition of two newcomers shifted the atmosphere. Then our friend came in and integrated us into the environment.

I tell you this story because it brings up two components of situational awareness—atmospherics and survival based on those atmospherics.

Atmospherics

Pay attention to the feel of any group or environment you find yourself in. People and moods can change abruptly.

Atmospherics is a distinct element of situational awareness. It includes the collective mood of the people, places, and things in your vicinity. It's reading the room and making changes to how you react based on the atmosphere.

Think about Maslow's hierarchy of needs. The biggest two are physiological needs followed by safety needs. Both of these are responses to, and demand that we pay attention to, our environment.

When we approached the backwoods building, the mood inside was celebratory. Everyone stopped, stared, and fell quiet when we entered. The mood swung to suspicion, a nonverbal "Why are you here? You don't belong."

When our friend came in and introduced us, everyone relaxed, and the atmosphere shifted back to celebration.

Maintaining awareness of disruptions in your environment is a must. But you live in a time when your needs are subsidized by and dependent on external systems, so your everyday experience doesn't teach that awareness organically.

Learning to notice and read the disruption in atmospherics among people and nature is critical to survival. I'm here to provide the atmospherics lessons you should have learned in your youth.

Baseline Summary

As the overall indicator of a situation, atmosphere contains many indicators:

- Physiological responses (biometrics)
- Body language and nonverbal communication (kinesics)
- Forms of contact between individuals (haptics)
- Interpersonal distances (proxemics)
- Physical signs, displays, and signals that convey meaning within the space (iconography)
- The level and types of noises present or missing
- Activity levels and forms of activity
- Levels of order and/or disorder
    - The difference between a march and a riot
    - Broken-window phenomenon: any sign of disorder leads to more disorder
    - Shopping cart theory: the number of misplaced shopping carts indicates an area's level of disorder

Atmospheric Anomalies

Any of these require immediate attention and represent a thread to pull on.

- Negative atmosphere
- Mismatched individual: a person deviating significantly from the situation's baseline
- Sudden change in mood

Source of Atmospheric Shifts: Positive, Negative, Neutral

When an atmospheric shift occurs, it is in response to something being added or removed from the environment.

- Response to the introduction of something enjoyable
- Response to presence of threat
- Response to authority

What caused the atmospheric shift? Be aware that it might be you.

Collective Mood

Atmospherics is experienced as a feeling, but there are definable indicators that inform its expression.

Emotions are honest. They are driven by subconscious autonomic processes that trigger before our conscious minds fit them into patterns. Others mimic those responses and patterns. Emotions can spread through a situation or environment to create a collective mood.

Survival Needs

Situational awareness using atmospherics helps us survive environments that turn hostile, even if they are beyond our control.

Maslow's hierarchy of needs demands we "read the room" and reorient our behavior as needed for our own well-being.

Some places are quiet; some are louder. But every environment has a baseline noise level. You should always be aware of it. Let me explain why.

After I got out of the service, I went to a bachelor party. We were at the bar listening to music, having some drinks, and hitting on girls. Those factors set the baseline atmospherics.

All of a sudden, hostile shouts mixed with the sounds of partying. I recognized one voice as belonging to a loudmouth friend of mine. Without knowing what he'd gotten himself into, I had to assume I was guilty by association. That meant I had to take action: confront the situation or abandon the people I was with.

It was scuffle stance time.

I hate bar fights. There are too many uncontrolled variables. And people get weird when they're drinking. I always assume every bar brawl has the potential to turn fatal.

My other more-or-less sober friends and I said, "Come on, guys, we're here for a bachelor party. This is supposed to be fun."

Everybody decided they'd rather enjoy a bachelor party than go to the ER, so we managed to de-escalate. Awareness of baseline atmospherics saved the party and maybe some lives.

How Atmospherics Relates to Baseline

Atmospherics and baseline (Chapter 4) are not different concepts; they are different levels of depth. As we dig deeper into the indicators that make up atmospherics, we will see that they are just additional indicators that form our baseline.

We're subject to atmospheric influence all the time. Think of standing in an elevator. You pick up everybody else's baseline behavior and start mimicking it.

But we're seldom conscious of that response. Increasing social awareness heightens your perception of atmospheric influences.

The Amygdala and Trusting Your Gut

The amygdala is the brain structure within your limbic system responsible for controlling your response to emotions and threats. When you say that you trust your gut, what you're doing is trusting your amygdala.

I'll teach you to interpret what your amygdala is telling you. That way, you can develop your amygdala to be trustworthy instead of acting on blind hunches.

Picking Up the Mood

Your amygdala lets you pick up on others' emotions by observing their physical state and their behavior. With it, you can feel the mood before checking the atmospherics for baseline anomalies.

Moods are contagious. As social animals, we have evolved to read the mood of the larger group. We are so good at it that we can do it over Zoom calls.

Because survival is prioritized over happiness, we have evolved a negative bias in our mood mimicry. Negative shifts in the atmospherics move faster through a group than positive ones.

Imagine you're at a restaurant. A man gets down on one knee. The whole restaurant gets excited and expectant. The man doesn't announce he's going to propose, yet everyone within eyeshot takes on the mood of expectation and excitement. When the woman says yes, the whole place cheers.

Now imagine the same couple arguing. They get louder and louder. The tables within earshot fall quiet. The whole restaurant becomes uncomfortable. When the woman stomps off, everyone in her path averts their eyes.

That illustrates how we pick on the collective mood of a situation or environment.

People have walked into armed robberies because they didn't pay attention to the atmospherics and didn't trust their amygdala. Lack of situational awareness has gotten people shot.

What do you expect to see when you walk into a gas station? The regular cashier greeting you with a friendly smile. A deliveryman restocking the refrigerator case. Customers playing on their phones while waiting to check out. That's your baseline.

Now imagine you go into the same gas station expecting your baseline, but someone is in the cashier's face. There are fewer shoppers than normal, and they all look tense. They stare at their shoes with terror on their faces.

This is why spotting anomalies in baselines is fundamental. But it's not the whole of situational awareness, just the introduction.

Noticing nonverbal behaviors is also key. The mood changes when your boss enters the break room. But that's normal, so it's the baseline. Everyone's behavior and nonverbal communication changes, even though no anomaly is present.

Atmospherics in Nature

We've covered the concept of the collective mood. Now let's discuss another important survival skill: understanding nature.

Picture this: you're hiking with your family. All of a sudden, you stop hearing the birds and insects. That's an atmospheric shift. It has nothing to do with people, but it still represents an anomaly in that environment.

Is the anomaly a weather change or a predator? In a survival context, identifying atmospherics relating to animals is critical to survival.

Seeing the Signs

Sign: any change in the natural state of an environment caused by animals, man, or machines.

Animals share the same basic needs we have, like food, water, and shelter. This means animals behave in predictable ways just like we do. So we can use their behavior to help us acquire resources.

You can observe animal behavior even when animals themselves aren't visible because animals leave trails.

Trails

Look for the following signs to find a trail:

- Displacement
- Stains
- Weathering
- Odor
- Litter

Displacement

Anything that has been moved from its original position, such as flattened plants, pressed-down rocks, or debris that's been pushed out of the path counts as displacement.

Displacements can be permanent, like snapped branches, or temporary, like trampled grass. Temporary displacements indicate how long ago something moved through the area. For instance, it takes a few minutes for short grasses to spring back up, longer for taller grasses.

How do you spot grass disruptions? Stepping on grass changes how it reflects the sun. You see it in how football fields and golf courses are mowed. Grass lying away from you looks light. Grass lying toward you is dark. So if an animal is moving away from you, the grass will be lighter.

Stains

Anything that discolors the natural setting, such as blood on leaves, mud on trees, or wetness in a dry environment, is a stain. Like displacements, stains can be permanent or temporary.

You know mud doesn't walk itself onto stones. If you see sand or mud on top of stones and it hasn't rained, you know something moved those materials.

Weathering

Weather effects also reveal the passage of time. If a snapped branch has dry leaves, you know it was broken some time ago.

Water washes signs away but also helps preserve them. A foot will leave a clearer print in wet sand. You can also tell if a disturbance occurred before or after it rained.

Wind moves things. If grass lies opposite the wind's direction, something pushed it in that direction. All these effects ought to be considered when evaluating trail indications.

Odor

Many animals have distinct scents. So do you. These can be followed if they are recent. Consider things like smoke, tobacco, and colognes. Anything that introduces a scent into the environment makes it easier to follow and identify a trail.

Litter

Leavings like food scraps or feces are litter. Feces will help identify what animal made the trail and how recently it passed through the area. Partially eaten and dropped seeds, seed pods, and carcasses are also animal identifiers. Of course, watch out for trash left by passing people.

Exercise

Find a patch of grass and walk through it. Circle around and look at the changes you caused.

Evading Predators

Animals don't pass through solid objects. They take the path of least resistance. Keep in mind, an animal's definition of "path of least resistance" differs from yours. A chain-link fence is an obstacle to you but not to a rabbit or a squirrel.

That said, taking the path of least resistance can make it easier for predators to predict your movements. Here's an example.

I grew up in rough neighborhoods. One night when I was fifteen, I was riding my skateboard home from a friend's house. The street lights came on as it got darker. Suddenly, a car full of older kids slammed on the brakes half a block away from me. They shouted, "We're gonna get you!"

Not knowing if these guys were serious or if they just wanted to chase me, I assumed they were serious. I fled down an alley. They pursued in the car. This went on for a few minutes until my brain caught up and thought, *I gotta get myself out of the situation.*

While they chased me down alleys, I realized they could only follow where cars could go. But I could use gaps, buildings, and the natural environment to go places they couldn't.

However, they knew my natural paths, too. If they saw me go toward a street, they'd pull into that street. If they didn't see me, they'd go around to the alley behind that street. It was a cat-and-mouse game.

So I shouldered the skateboard, hopped fences, and cut through yards. I left all the natural paths and made one to evade the predators.

Being aware of my situation, knowing where predators could go, and understanding where they thought I could go saved me from whatever trouble my pursuers had in mind. To sum it all up, survival involves learning a few basic skills. Determine a baseline, spot anomalies, identify threats, and discover the resources available to you.

CHAPTER 7

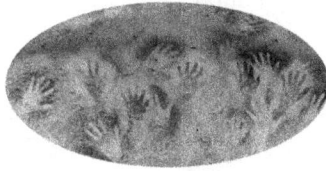

WATER: FIND IT, FILTER IT, DON'T DIE

Do you know how to get drinkable water? It's one of Maslow's level 1 needs, along with food and shelter. Most likely, your answer is to pour some from the faucet. But if society collapses, will you be able to find a steady source of water to ensure your survival?

After this chapter, you will. You'll know how to find and purify water out in the wild. And with these two fundamental survival skills, you'll know where to look for water and how to treat that water so it doesn't make you sick.

Being without water for an unsafe period of time is one of the worst experiences you can undergo. In my senior year in high school, I came down with appendicitis. I needed surgery to have my appendix removed. After a short hospital stay, I was discharged. But it turned out there were some complications from the surgery. I couldn't keep anything down for a week afterward.

It was miserable. I couldn't even keep water down. Dehydration set in after the third day. And by the fourth day, I had to go to the emergency room. The nursing staff couldn't even find a vein to start an IV. My condition worsened as they struggled to figure out a solution.

The nurses had to call in a medical student who'd been practicing on cadavers. She came in and found a shriveled but viable vein to get a needle into. Finally!

I survived severe dehydration, but it came down to the wire.

Many people don't realize that the sensation of thirst is a sign of dehydration. If you feel thirsty, you're not drinking enough.

Climate and activity aside, you can last about three days without water. I was past that mark when they put the IV in me, and I want to spare you that agony. Since finding water is a matter of life and death, even more so than getting food, we'll cover how to find water first.

Maybe you're saying, "That's easy. I'll just find a pond or a stream."

And you'd say that because people in the West take clean drinking water for granted. After all, it's on tap in all our homes. But that just means we're dependent on the city water supply or store-bought bottled water.

Even with current technology, it's hard to make water safe to drink. Modern sewage systems employ two levels of treatment. The first step uses a screen to catch large objects. After that, water flows into a grit chamber, which separates out stuff like sand. Then the water flow slows enough to let the remaining particles settle at the bottom of a sedimentation tank.

The next step uses one of two methods to remove about 85 percent of organic matter from the water. The first method involves filtering the sewage water through a bed of stones or corrugated plastic laden with bacteria. That bacteria break down the organic remnants, and cleaner water heads to another sedimentation tank that clears out the bacteria. Chemical disinfection, often with chlorine, comes next.

The second method is more common. Sludge—the remnants of organic matter—is introduced into the sewage, air is pumped into the chamber, and the whole mess is left to stew. Microorganisms in the bacteria-rich mixture break down the remaining organic matter in the half-treated sewage. The water is pumped out, and the sludge left over from this process gets recycled into the next batch of water. And, as in the first method, the newly cleaned water undergoes chemical disinfection.[3]

It's the disgusting miracle behind your clean and convenient water. And it's a young miracle. In the mid-1800s, the average adult male got the majority of his water from beer, the cleanest beverage to drink. In fact, up here in the Twin Cities, the local breweries offer to fill up jugs with spring water for free. They *had* to clean the water.

But in a survival situation, clean water won't be convenient. Tap water is given to you, but how do you get water for yourself?

First, you need to learn a new term. This will be the key to locating water no matter where you are in the world.

Your new best friend in a survival situation is the riparian zone.

What does that term mean? Let me explain . . .

Finding Water

Riparian zones are places where vegetation and the environment respond to the presence of water. They're the best places to live in any biome.

How do you find riparian zones? Be aware of shifts in the kinds of plants growing in your surroundings. Take the American sycamore tree; it's large and has white, peeling bark. And it lives near water.

Say you're walking through an evergreen forest, and you suddenly come into an area full of trees that look like sycamores or any deciduous trees. Because those trees require more water than evergreens, you've probably stumbled onto a zone with a water table near the surface.

And trees themselves can be sources of water. Have you ever cut a root and seen the tree bleed? Or seen a maple tree tapped to make syrup? Both tap into a tree's water lines. Trees use water to carry sap, and the sap carries nutrients from root to branch. That means you can cut a hole through the bark to get water.

---

3 - United States Environmental Protection Agency, Office of Water, "How Wastewater Treatment Works . . . The Basics," May 1998, https://www3.epa.gov/npdes/pubs/bastre.pdf.

Research plants in your local area to figure out which are the best to tap. Plants with overlapping leaves make natural funnels that gather water. You can also tap bamboo stalks like trees. Gourds in the ground have pulp you can scrape into your shirt and squeeze water from. You won't get a ton of water that way, but it's better than nothing.

The good news is you can find riparian zones anywhere, even in deserts. Wander a dry creek bed, and you'll see growth here and there. Those plants' taproots are digging down to water. You can do the same with simple tools or even your hands. Contrary to popular belief, you can't drink from a cactus. But it has waterlogged pulp inside you can scrape and press like a gourd's.

Plants aren't the only water sources in a riparian zone. Let me show you some more.

Terrain and Surface Water

Water you can see and hear is the easiest to find. This is surface water you can step in or even bathe in, like rivers, lakes, and streams. Even natural potholes and pockets of stones can collect rainwater. Look upstream for surface water's origin because springs are naturally filtered.

Water always wants to move downhill, so look in valleys, gullies, and ditches. Look for erosion patterns in the ground. These can point you to riparian zones.

You can also follow game trails and observe wildlife. Look for multiple converging trails and follow that larger trail. It will lead you to water. If you're following a trail that splits into smaller trails, you're probably moving away from water.

Most herd animals will head toward their water source at dusk and dawn. The same is true of seed-eating birds. Follow them. Also, bees never make a hive more than five kilometers or so from a water source.

What do you do when you find signs of a riparian zone but no visible water?

You dig.

Groundwater

Look for moss or algae. Dig nearby for groundwater held in an aquifer beneath the surface. Go an arm's length down, from shoulder to fingertip. If you don't hit water, move to a different spot. You're making what's called a seepage basin.

And if you dig down half that depth and it's dry, you're probably in a bad spot. The soil should get wetter as you go down. When you dig deep enough, water will start to seep in from the edges of your pit. Let it fill for a couple of hours, if you can afford to. This also allows the sediment you've dug up to settle.

The water won't seep back into the soil as long as the hole is below the water level. Gravity is your friend here. You want to find a low spot to start digging. If you have to dig more than five feet, you've started too high.

You can do the same with other water sources. Say you find a pond, but it's scummy. Or you're in a bog, marsh, or fen. You wouldn't want to touch it, much less drink it. So go about ten feet from the shoreline on dry land, and dig an arm's length down again. Since your hole is below the waterline, water will seep in and get filtered.

It works the same way with saltwater. If you're on an ocean shore, go inland just past the first dunes and dig your hole. You'll have enough tightly packed sand to start filtering the salt out of that water.

When you've found water, be careful before you drink it. Use your senses. Look around. Are there dead animals lying near the water source? Is the vegetation around it dying? Clean water has no odor. Does the water smell? All these are signs you may have a bad water source.

But when you find water, what do you do with it?

Filtering and Treating Water

Your seepage pit will start the process and remove some potential contaminants from the water. But you should filter and boil it whenever possible. Boiling is the number one way to kill anything alive in the water.

In the 1870s, when dysentery would sweep through railroad worker camps, the Chinese laborers wouldn't get sick. Others accused them of poisoning the water, but they were just boiling it to make tea. This killed off the bacteria in their water supply and rendered it safe to drink.

If you're in an emergency situation and you think rescue is likely, you can risk diarrhea and vomiting from drinking unboiled water. It might keep you alive long enough to be rescued. But this book isn't concerned about survival rescue situations. I want to give you the skill set to make water safe to consume as needed.

First, you should know how to build filters. There are a few ways to do this, but they all use the same basic elements.

The Three-Part Water Filter You Can Make Yourself

The first step is finding a vessel to hold water. If you can scrounge one up, great. If not, you can use hollow logs or curved pieces of bark.

You could also make a burn bowl. Start a fire, and get a large enough piece of wood. Heap coals on the area of that wood you want to hollow into a bowl. After the coals burn through part of the wood, dump them out and use a sharp stone to scrape out the burned layer beneath. This will take a while, and you will have to repeat this process several times to make it as deep as you need it.

You'll need two vessels for this method. Start by filling one with water. Then stretch your shirt or another piece of cloth over the empty vessel's opening. Put rocks over the shirt so it dips down a bit. Then pour water through the cloth membrane slowly. You don't want to lose any, if possible.

This first bulk filter will remove anything bigger than the pores of your cloth. Once you've run all the water through the filter, get rid of the rocks. Rinse your shirt as best you can, and shake it out. Now put it over the just-emptied container. Swapping back and forth between vessels could reintroduce some contaminants, but this is better than nothing.

Next, gather some sand, as fine grained as you can get, and pile it on the cloth. If you can't find sand, you can use dirt. Pour the stone-filtered water through the sand. Now take the sand off your shirt, rinse the cloth as best you can, and transfer the shirt to the now-empty vessel.

Time to use charcoal. We'll cover how to make it later. Charcoal is super porous, so water flows right through it, which helps remove toxic minerals, toxic chemicals, and other potential contaminants. Almost every water filter uses it, even the LifeStraw.

Crush the charcoal as fine as you can, and put it on the shirt. Pour the water through slowly like you did with the sand and rocks.

Now you've filtered your water. In fact, you've done it the same way emerging economies do long-term water treatments. They use a barrel of rocks, a barrel of sand, and a barrel of charcoal—in that order.

You can get creative with your filters. Stack the same ingredients in a two-liter bottle with the rocks on top where you pour the water in, charcoal on the bottom where the water comes out. Separate the layers with cloth in between. You can even build the same filter in a sock!

Once your water is filtered, you'll need to boil and purify it. But first, let's go over how to make charcoal.

How and Why to Make Charcoal

Charcoal is not *burned* wood; it is *cooked* wood with all the moisture and gasses removed. It's different from ash, though both charcoal and ash can be handy. In fact, you can use both to make sure your digestive system is working right. If you're constipated, add a little bit of ash to your water and drink it. If you have diarrhea, add a little bit of charcoal. Just remember: "White if you're tight, black if you're loose."

The charcoal we're talking about isn't the kind you get from a store in a Kingsford bag. That stuff has additives. If you go to a barbecue or smoker store, they'll have something called lump charcoal. That is what we're talking about: just cooked wood, a brick of pure carbon.

To make charcoal, you introduce high heat to the wood at low oxygen so the wood doesn't become fuel. You can pull some charcoal out of most campfires, but we want to make it intentionally. Here are a few ways to do it.

The mound method involves stacking wood, preferably hard wood, close together. Put the largest and thickest pieces in the middle with the smaller pieces toward the outside. Pile mud and dirt on the stack, but leave one hole on top and eight holes around the bottom. Light the fire at the top, and when it reaches one of the bottom holes, seal it with mud.

Repeat this process until all eight holes are covered, and then seal the top with mud. If you see any cracks forming, cover them with mud, too. Leave the mound to cool, which may take a few days. Then crack it open to find the charcoal.

You can also use a metal can, like a paint can. Pack the can as full of wood as you're able, since you want as little oxygen in there as possible. Again, you want to cook the wood, not burn it. Once the can is packed, seal it with the lid. Poke a hole in the top so pressure can escape. Then put the can in a fire. Smoke will come out of the hole. Some of that smoke might be a substance called wood gas, which may catch fire, so be careful.

When smoke and gas stop coming out of the ventilation hole, the can is ready. Plug the hole to keep stray sparks or flames from igniting the charcoal, and let the can cool. Once it cools enough to handle, open it up to find your charcoal.

How and Why to Purify Water

The way to purify water in a survival situation is to boil it with rocks.

We'll cover making fire in a later chapter. For now, let's assume you have a lighter or some other fire source. We'll also assume you don't have a pot to cook it in, and you're using a natural container like a hollowed-out log.

First, fill your container with the water you filtered earlier. Then get a fire going. Put some rocks in the fire, and let them get hot. Then use a couple of sticks as tongs to move the rocks from the fire to your container of water. Keep rotating hot rocks in and out until the water boils. You can also use this technique to cook soup.

Bring the water to a rolling boil for about ten minutes. You can boil it for less time at lower elevations, but no matter where you are, boiling for ten minutes will kill everything in the water.

Let the water cool from a boil. Wait about as long as you would before drinking tea. It won't be cold like bottled spring water, but it'll be drinkable.

There are other ways to purify water. You can use chemical tablets, like iodine or chlorine. Make sure to follow the EPA guidelines, or you risk making the water undrinkable. Other products, like the LifeStraw, can be used to purify water, but you have to follow the manufacturer's instructions.

Depending on your water source, you needn't always use all these steps. If you can find a clean spring coming right out of the ground, you *probably* don't have to filter it. You should be able to consume rainwater directly, but there's always a risk.

Why boil water? Because there might be contaminants in the ground. Or a dead animal upstream might be releasing all kinds of bacteria into the water, which is why it's also a good idea to head upstream and see where the water is coming from. Even rainwater might have pollutants that need to be cleaned out.

Just remember that boiling water is guaranteed to kill anything living in there. It never hurts to filter water, either. If you're not on the verge of dying from thirst, boil the water. If it's life or death, you can risk drinking it. But some stuff you should never drink.

What Not to Drink and Why

One thing you do *not* want to do is drink urine. Normal urine is 95 percent water, but by the time you're dehydrated enough to consider drinking pee, the concentrations of toxins and salts will be closer to 30 percent. If you drink that, your body will have to use its own water to eliminate the salt from your system. Drinking urine will remove water from your body, creating a negative feedback loop.

Blood is likewise high in sodium and has plasmas and other substances your body must use water to process out. And of course, don't drink salt water for the same reason.

Don't eat snow, either. Your body will have to burn calories to keep your temperature up. Instead, melt it back into water first. If you have a fire going, gather snow in a piece of cloth and bring it near enough to the fire that it starts to melt. Put a container underneath to collect the meltwater. If you don't have a fire but you have a water bottle, add some snow to the water already inside and put it inside your clothing for your body heat to melt.

Once the snow is melted, the same rules for rainwater apply. If you live in an area with high pollution, it's best to filter and purify. But if you live in an area where you can drink the rainwater, you can drink melted snow. Snow is just cold rainwater. It's less likely to have anything living in it because it's frozen. And there shouldn't be many bacteria, viruses, or protozoa falling from the sky. The evaporation process takes care of them.

You have several options for collecting water, but they often require access to specific materials. Preppers favor using plastic bags to capture dew off trees. You can cut a hole in the bag and tie it around a branch so the hole is on the bottom. But who carries plastic bags around?

Another option is using solar distilleries. You dig a hole in sand or dirt, spread some vegetation on the bottom, and put a cup in the middle. Then cover with a clear plastic tarp, and put a stone in the middle to dip downward over the cup. Water will evaporate from the vegetation at the bottom of the pit and condense on the bottom of the plastic sheet. Gravity will make it drip into the cup.

The one problem with a solar distillery is that you need clear plastic. Carrying around a plastic bag is not a skill. But being able to find and filter your own water is.

Products like the LifeStraw are great if you have them, but they wear out. That's why I don't call myself a prepper. Preppers have rooms full of food. But what happens when the food runs out? They have boxes full of bullets. But what happens when the ammo's spent? What do you do when somebody sets your house on fire and forces you to abandon your stores?

You have to fall back on a skill set—the same skill set your ancestors used to survive a world trying to kill them.

What Next?

The first thing you should do is learn to identify what your local riparian zone looks like. Research which plants live there. Take a walk by a local creek to see what's growing there and not growing anywhere else.

And try out some of these skills. Build a water filter out of the sock whose match the dryer ate. Crush up some charcoal, and put it in the bottom of the sock. If you have a bit of cloth or even some of the cordage you processed, ball that up to form a barrier the water can pass through and stuff it on top of the charcoal.

Then throw some fine sand on top of the cloth barrier. Add another permeable barrier, throw the rocks on top of it, and you've got a three-part filter in a sock!

Next, go find some water. Dig down below the water table, and let some water collect. Then pour it into the top of your filter, and let it seep all the way through. The stuff that comes out the bottom will be filtered water. The sock's sides will leak, but depending on the material, it will swell as it gets damp. The wetter it gets, the more it'll keep water on the inside because the gaps in the fabric will close.

If you've got a small cast-iron skillet, put it over a fire you've made. Boil the filtered water for ten minutes, let it cool, and drink it. You just found, gathered, filtered, and consumed water you made safe by your own hand!

Next, you'll learn how to read your surroundings for signs of danger.

CHAPTER 8

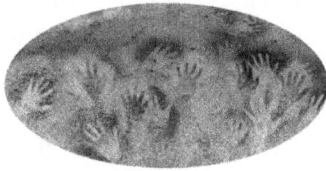

PROXEMICS: GIVE YOURSELF MORE THAN TWO SECONDS TO REACT

Running my tongue across my top row of teeth, I tasted metallic, salty blood. I wanted to spit it out but denied my opponent the satisfaction. The two of us held eye contact. The beginnings of a smile tugged the corners of my mouth upward. I sucked in a breath through my nose. It wasn't time to piss him off, not just yet.

We moved in close. His arm snaked around my neck. My hand pushed down on his chest. One of us was going down; who depended on one question: What's more important, training or sheer force?

Marine basic hand-to-hand combat training was grueling. Our enemy wouldn't hold back in war, so why should we in training? We all wanted to be the best. It wasn't about ego. It was about instilling the ability to evaluate a problem and overcome it in the face of fear. No one benefited from being treated with kid gloves, so the gloves were off.

Drill instructor Gunnery Sergeant Maitland was tough but fair. He had the ability to match us with challenging opponents. It was as if he could see each recruit's weakness and find a sparring partner who could exploit that vulnerability. The rules were simple: don't break any bones, and fight until the drill instructor tells you to stop.

My sparring buddy was a semipro boxer with eight wins, two of them knockouts. We called him Larry the Lugger. He was stocky and strong, his footwork was fast, and he could hit hard. Imagine going up against a barrel on roller skates with a mean right hook.

I'd wrestled in high school six months of the year, but Larry boxed year round. If I could get close to him, I could put him on the ground and do some damage. But his southpaw swing could keep me at bay. On paper, the smart money was on the shorter, stronger, better-trained guy. But if I've taught you anything so far, it's that the map is not the territory.

When Larry and I were first paired up, I prepared myself to get whipped. But then I was given an advantage: one variable that shifted the odds back to even.

The combat arena.

A four-by-four square was all we had. It may not seem like a big deal, but having to fight in close quarters eliminated all Larry's advantages. Without room for him to float like a butterfly, I dropped him like a rock. And once I had him on the ground where his training was worthless, he panicked. I pinned him, and he tapped out.

The next time we fought, he adapted his strategy. Instead of treating it like a boxing match, he became a mad dog, doing whatever he could to win. We fought several bouts that left us both with bloody noses and black eyes.

I would love to say that I won most of the time. But put it like this: I won more times than I should have.

Larry and I bonded over trading punches and became friends. Sometimes it happens that way. Each of us wanted to be the best so we could rely on each other in a foxhole. We both rose to the challenge, and I'm grateful to him. Being forced to fight in close quarters turned what should've been a clear victory for the boxer into a series of draws for the wrestler. It goes to show that a factor like proximity made all the difference.

they were from the equator, the more they kept their distance. But these variations still fall within four zones of proximity. They are:

- Intimate Zone (0″–18″): Close relations. The highest risk with immediate exposure to deadly force.
- Personal Zone (18″–4′): Friends and acquaintances. High risk still in immediate exposure to deadly force.
- Social Zone (4′–10′): Strangers you may have a reason to engage with (giving a presentation). Risk of exposure to deadly force, out of direct contact but compromising your reaction window.
- Public Zone (10′–25′): Strangers that must be acknowledged and are on your radar. Risk of exposure to deadly force, out of direct contact but compromising your reaction window.

People outside the public zone will not be on your radar. You may be aware of them, but you won't consider them a threat.

Imagine you're walking down a crowded street. Someone comes through the crowd from the opposite direction, bumping and bouncing off everyone. Why would someone be violating other people's intimate space? This is where context comes into play. How is the oncomer moving? Is this individual staggering with arms flailing? It could be a drunk. Is this person hunched over, hand to mouth, glancing back every couple of seconds? That person could be fleeing someone or something.

If you live in a big city, you're never more than two seconds away from danger. There's always someone in your public zone. If you factor in variables like time of day, how well the street is lit, and the absence of security cameras or other people, the potential for harm multiplies. All it takes is one person ready to risk those two seconds.

But proximity makes you more able to pick up on subtle cues from people. Look at them and read their body language. Does the person seem tense? That rigidity could signal mental preparation to take action.

Picture yourself in a bar talking to a pretty blonde in a blue dress. Out of the corner of your eye, you see a large silhouette appear in the bright white light coming from the bathroom. The shape is headed in your and the blonde's direction. All you can see are two unblinking eyes locked on you. Does the context and his closing proximity indicate he randomly selected you to pursue? Or is it more likely you are hitting on his partner?

Proxemics isn't just about how people move. It's about the context in which they move. The environment can help predict behavior. We perform many subconscious actions. Consider the humble elevator. You get in on the ground floor and punch the button for the thirtieth floor. It goes up a floor and stops. Another traveler embarks. What happens next? That's right, you both move to the other side of the car. Then it gets worse; a third person enters. The two of you move to the back and give the front area to the third. Somehow you knew to do that without being told.

If you want to have some fun the next time you get into a crowded elevator, instead of facing the doors like a sane person, face the crowd. See how long you can last before they call in the SWAT team.

While proxemics deals with the subtleties and nuance of human inter-action, it can also encompass basic safety needs. How close you are to shelter or water will affect your behavior and the behavior of your group.

Push versus Pull

It's a hot summer's day. Kids are playing in the park. They shout as they tumble and try to go the whole way around on the swing. One of the kids hears something and stops. The kid goes to the edge of the park and stands at the sidewalk, looking left and right. Another child steps away from the seesaw and joins the first at the sidewalk. Then another child, and another and another. Before you know it, the park is empty, and there is a crowd of kids standing with expectant looks on their faces.

Then you hear it: the jingle of the ice cream truck.

An attractor stimulus, like the ice cream truck above, is a pull prox-emic. It doesn't even have to be an incentive. You've seen a car crash on the opposite side of the freeway and slowed down to rubberneck. The event is pulling you in like a magnet.

But magnets can attract and repel. Think back to what you did when a group of people were running in your direction. There's a good chance you ran with them without thinking. Sometimes the threat may be so close, you have no time to think, and your animal instinct kicks in.

We are pack animals at the end of the day. For all our intelligence and sophistication, it does not always take much to spook us. Sometimes it's for the best, but this is why it is always good to be aware of your surroundings. The proxemic push-pull is always giving us hints about what is going on in the immediate environment.

But that's not the only way to look at proxemics.

Marking Your Territory

Proxemics is also a way to mark your territory. The three types of static territory are primary, secondary, and public.

Primary territory relates to where you live. These are places like your room, your house, or your car. In fact, another term for it is *home territory*. You have continuous control over your primary territory. You're at your most comfortable there, and if someone enters that area without your consent, it feels like a violation.

Secondary territory is interactional. This is an area where you expect to see the same people consistently. The best example of this would be your workplace. You view parts of it as "yours" but understand that parts of it belong to others. If you work in an office, you expect to see coworkers, bosses, secretaries, and security guards. There are expectations of dress code and behavior. For example, you cannot run around the office with your pants down, shouting, "I'm a zebra!" At least not for long.

The final territory, public, is a space that is open and accessible to anyone. Almost anyone can go to a public park or a movie theater. And this is where the twenty-five-foot rule comes into play.

It's important to keep in mind that what is a primary territory for you might be a secondary territory for another. The cubicle in your office may be your primary territory, but your boss won't look at it the same way. He views it as secondary, and someone from outside the office might view it as public.

Now think about proxemics in a survival setting. Say you come up against a warlord who views a local water source as primary territory, and you view it as public. Who's right? Do you potentially risk your life and challenge him, or do you find somewhere else to drink? These are crucial decisions that you may have to make. Our proxemic decisions today may be more nuanced than this, but they are driven by the same forces.

And be aware of territorial markers. We want to protect our territory, so we mark it with objects or, in some cases, our bodies. In a civilized society, there are subtle means of signifying your space. While waiting for a friend in a crowded cafe, you may drape a coat over a stool to nonverbally communicate, "This spot is taken." That's known as a central marker.

The second type is a boundary marker. It's a fence, a gate, or other object that lets you know that the territory beyond the marker is not yours.

The third territorial marker claims something as yours. Labeling your lunch or personalizing your car with bumper stickers are two examples. Both tell others, "This is mine. Hands off."

Problems arise when people cannot respect boundaries. Let's look at an example next.

(Un)Clear and Present Danger

There had been a rise in unprovoked attacks in cities. No one is safe. The viral social media sensation called the knockout game involved an accomplice filming a perpetrator assaulting a passerby at random. Actor Rick Moranis was sucker punched by a homeless man in 2020.

It's not limited to physical violence. Think of all the metropolitan areas you've been to that have signs reading WARNING: PICKPOCKETS OPERATE IN THIS AREA.

Those are just the threats posed by your fellow humans. Vehicles, open sewer grates, and debris falling from buildings can be just as hazardous. Either way, you have twenty-five feet and two seconds to respond.

Twenty-five feet is the distance from one side of the street to the other. Things could turn nasty in an eyeblink. That's why you have to be aware of your surroundings at all times.

What should you do if someone comes at you? Your options are fight, flight, or freeze. Most people will freeze. Some will flee; take that option if you can, no matter the nature of the threat. It's not like the movies where the henchmen take turns fighting the hero. You want to get outside that twenty-five-foot range and keep it that way. If you can, run toward other people, even just two or three. There is safety in numbers, and if you're being chased by a mugger, one witness may save your wallet.

A Word about Cell Phones

Imagine your friend builds a time machine, and you go back to the caveman days. You see some people in stylish saber-toothed tiger skins. You keep your Zippo in your pocket and pretend to be fascinated by the fire they just invented.

You grunt your goodbyes, get back in the time machine, and head back to present day. But something's not right. Instead of Times Square, you find nothing but grassland. You realize you made a mistake and hop back in the time machine. And you find the blankets empty and the fire out. In place of the cavemen, there's a saber-toothed tiger with blood on his fangs.

Meowing comes from a light in the middle of the clearing. It's not the tiger's cubs. It's the phone you realize you left behind. You doomed the human race with cat videos.

We're not much more advanced than our cave-dwelling ancestors. Our instincts and gut feelings all come from them. Technology has exploded, and we've been caught in the fallout from the internet. A smartphone is a vortex of distractions and spatial obliviousness. How many near misses have you had with someone whose face was buried in a phone? How many times have you almost walked into someone who was too absorbed in texting?

Make a habit of noticing what's twenty-five feet away from you at all times. Integrate it into your routine. Learn to do it on a regular basis, and you'll put yourself ahead of the pack. You'll be able to see farther ahead and plan accordingly.

CHAPTER 9

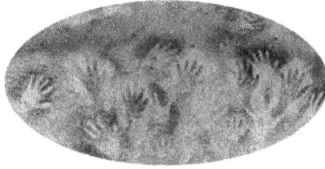

NOT-SO-FAST FOOD: HUNTING AND GATHERING FOR PEOPLE WHO DIDN'T GROW UP DOING EITHER

Before you read on, know that things get a little less pleasant going forward. Because life isn't always pretty, but you'll want to know what to do when it gets ugly.

When it comes to survival, you will have to do things you're not comfortable with. Few people these days are familiar with hunting and gathering. In this chapter, we'll be covering snaring and skinning game.

It's not that I revel in cruelty. It's that survival means tapping into primal instincts. Early humans did whatever they could to survive, and their survival depended on not starving to death. Yours does, too. That means keeping your strength up, and that means getting your protein.

Meat is rich in protein. And meat is found in animals. We'll get into plant-based protein sources for vegetarians and vegans, but understand that wild plants come with higher risks.

If you want to survive, you have to make mature decisions. If you'd rather starve than kill a squirrel, that's fine. Lie down and die on principle. But what if it wasn't just you? Maybe you're stranded with an older or younger relative. Maybe you're comfortable with dying for your beliefs, but are you comfortable with making someone else die for them? What if you make it out, and your loved one doesn't? Could you live with that?

I'm not here to convince you to eat meat. What you put into your body is your choice. What I am trying to teach you is that surviving may mean doing things you never thought you were capable of. Nature isn't nice. If you want to survive, you can't be nice, either.

Weekends with Dad

When I was growing up, my parents seldom shared the same house, let alone the same room. They married and divorced twice, but they had enough of a mutual attraction to have three kids together.

I was the oldest. Dad struggled with alcoholism and drug addiction throughout my childhood. My brothers and I didn't see him much. He wanted to make the one weekend a month we spent together eventful, so he'd take us to some historic sites. Or we'd go digging for dinosaur bones in sandstone quarries.

Dad liked being outdoors, away from the city. He'd been a camp counselor when he was younger, so he was used to sleeping under the stars. My brothers and I brought tents. Dad said he took us camping every month to keep us out of harm's way. But sometimes I wonder if it was to keep him out of trouble, too.

Dad took a live-off-the-land approach to feeding us. On the occasions we went camping with him, the rule was we could only eat what we could catch.

Dad's favorite form of hunting was fishing. I can still see him, standing in the sunset with his line in his hand down by the lake. If you are stranded in the wilderness with no other food, you will need to hunt. Having my dad teach me even the little he did was invaluable. So let me teach you.

The Hunt Is On

Hunting is the capture of live animals as a food source. This discipline brings together many of the skills you've been developing in the previous chapters.

You may not want to hunt. You may not even want to eat meat. But vegetarianism and veganism are luxuries for when things are going well. Do you think primal man had the luxury of choice?

Our ancestors' only choice was feast or famine. And if it was famine, keep in mind, it only takes a few short knocks to the supply chain before you're back to the same level as your primitive forebears. Maybe you bought this book because you saw how fast things can go south, and you wanted to be better equipped for emergencies.

Knowing how to hunt is the most essential skill for keeping you alive. What kinds of game can you hunt? Read on to find out.

The Three Fs of Hunting and Gathering

If it has fur, feathers, or fins and you can catch, clean, and cook it, there's a low chance that eating it will kill you. Some animals, like the lionfish, are poisonous. But the three Fs are good guides for choosing what to hunt.

Hunting comes in two forms—active and passive. Here's the difference.

Passive Hunting versus Active Hunting

Passive is low risk with no skills required. You won't have to exert yourself much. The only aspect to keep in mind is you need to know where the prey will be.

- **Active** has more potential risk. You'll need training to a certain degree of skill. You'll already know where the prey is, but catching it will take a considerable energy investment.

Passive Hunting: Snaring Rabbits and Hares

Rabbits and hares make good target animals for teaching purposes because they're widely available year round. The steps will be similar for any small mammal.

Steps to Snaring

1. Find the game trail.

Your first step to snaring is to find a game trail. When you're collecting water or wood for your shelter, you may discover one by chance. If you want to seek one out, there are a few options.

Remember that other mammals have the same needs as you: food, water, and shelter. For now, forget about where they source their food because, like you, they won't always get it from one spot. You'll just waste energy trying to find them there.

Where they find water and shelter will be more consistent. For small animals, keep your eyes peeled for holes in the ground and tree hollows, which are more likely to be sleep locations. Once you have found the bedding area, you can search for a game trail.

But water sources are your best bet. A given area will only have one main water source. It could be a lake, a river, a stream, or even a pond. Animals will be there at least once a day. If you search along the waterline, you have a high chance of finding a game trail. And the wet ground will make it easier to pick up the tracks.

Once you have found the game trail, look for a bottleneck. That's where you should set up your snare.

2: Set up the snare.

The most simple snare you can create is a cordage snare. Making one will require using your cordage-making skills, like so:

- Bend six inches of cord back on itself.
- Tie this loop into an overhand knot, leaving a loop after the knot.
- Bend the loop back on itself.
- Run the cordage tail through loop eyelets and across or behind the knot side of the loop.

Once complete, attach the snare to a solid object like a rooted plant or stake it to the ground.

Build up the constriction around the snare. This will increase the odds of the prey running into the snare. Add material on either side, and push a small stick into the ground below the snare. That encourages the target animal to raise its head as it goes through the snare.

You'll need to make more than one snare. Make sure to set several along as many game paths as you can find.

Once you have set them, check the snares regularly. Other animals will take advantage of captured prey. Do not lose your catch to them!

Field Dressing Rabbits and Hares

Leaving the carcass intact increases the potential for harmful bacteria to develop, so dress the catch as soon as you can after it has died.

Complete Dress

Here are the step-by-step instructions you'll need.

1. Make a cut across the midback.
2. Work the fingers of opposite hands into both sides of this cut and pull the fur and skin off like you are peeling off a tight pair of socks.
3. Remove the feet.
4. Remove the head.
5. Find the sternum. Just below it, make a shallow cut into the chest cavity toward the heart.
6. Being careful, slice the abdomen open from sternum to tail. Cut around the anus.
    a. You can use your fingers to separate the membrane from the innards as you slice to make sure you don't open the bladder or intestines.
7. Crack the rib cage open.
8. Hold the carcass vertically, and take care to separate the connective tissue around the heart and lungs from the body. Then pull the innards out.
9. Check the liver and other organs.
    a. White spots on the liver indicate potential illness, and the animal ought to be discarded.
    b. Look for any other signs of illness in the organs such as discoloration, a stink, or parasites. If in doubt, chuck it out.
10. Discard feet, head, and innards.
11. Cut the rear legs at the hip joint, and snap the joint apart to separate.
12. Cut the front legs at the shoulder, and snap the shoulder joint apart to separate.
13. Cut the loin from along the spine.
14. Cook the meat thoroughly.

Passive Hunting: Fish Trap

Here we will set up a static fish trap that can be used to catch aquatic animals. This method works best in freshwater areas.

Materials

You will need a couple of dozen rigid arm-length sticks. You'll also need as much pliable material like roots, grass, or stalks as you can carry to the site of your trap.

Trap Steps

Follow these steps in order and without skipping any.

1. Find a corner or bend in a creek, stream, or river. If you're hunting a larger body of water, such as a pond or lake, look for a natural pocket in the shoreline. You want this area to form the walls of your trap as much as possible, so the narrower the pocket or bend, the better.
2. Pound the rigid sticks into the ground across the opening of the bend or pocket to make a funnel. Place the large end facing the body of water and the small end facing into your bend or pocket.
   a. Think of this as making a connect-the-dots pattern in the form of a funnel.
   b. Weave the pliable roots, stalks, and grasses in and out of the rigid sticks on either side of the funnel mouth.
3. Try to use the most flexible materials nearest the small mouth of the funnel. These will bow in slightly and make it harder for captured animals to leave the trap.
4. You will end up with two separate walls that mirror each other forming the shape of a funnel.
5. Toss the remaining loose material into the water of the trap to create a natural shade spot to attract animals.

6. Bait the trap. Use leftovers from the rabbit or hare you caught or anything else you can find.
7. If you have no bait, find a branch that has many smaller branches. Use it to agitate the water downstream to scare fish into the trap. This works best in smaller streams and creeks.

Gather

Hunting and gathering go hand in hand. As you set snares and traps, be alert for edible plants, sources of cordage materials, new game trails, and shelters.

Gathering will be an ongoing activity. Whenever you move through an environment, view it as a general store. What do they have on the shelves? Is there anything on sale (i.e., is it easy to acquire)?

Situational awareness is the skill of evaluating our environment. Gathering is the skill of recognizing useful materials in the environment.

Never Stop Eating

Gathering food is an essential skill, even when you're feeling more confident about passive hunting. Anytime you find yourself without immediate access to food, you're at risk of going hungry.

Hunting requires factors you're not always in control of: the prey, mainly. You may find that other predators have slipped in and stolen your dinner. That's why you should always be eating when you're in the wilderness. But you need to learn how to recognize what is and is not a food source.

The crucial factor in using plants as food is not poisoning yourself.

Most people are unfamiliar with plants. Some will feed you while others will kill you. And some plants appear similar to others, but they have subtle differences. It's important to know those differences. Gathering is a process of elimination. Remove any potential food that may cause you harm.

Your best option is to learn in advance which plants in your local area are edible. Most people spend much of their lives in the same or similar areas. Learning which local plants are safe to eat would be easy. But they don't seek that knowledge because they think they'll never need it. Learning from those who have already done the testing can save you time, broaden your options, and spare you major discomfort.

Whether you're already familiar with wild plants or you are testing a new one, eat them in moderation. Plants can affect people in different ways. And even if they're edible, they can still cause distress if consumed in large quantities.

Read on to save yourself the pain of learning the hard way.

Avoid the Following

Plants growing along roadsides or near heavily occupied buildings

- Plants growing in contaminated water
- Plants with obvious signs of fungal growth
- Plants with milky or discolored sap
- Plants with a bitter or soapy taste
- Plants with thorns, spines, or fine hairs
- Plants with dill-, carrot-, or parsley-type foliage
- Plants with an almondlike scent in their more woody parts
- Grain heads with pink, purple, or black spurs
- Plants with three-leaved growth patterns

And never eat mushrooms! Some mushrooms have symptoms that only show up days after ingestion, so mushrooms are not viable options for the Universal Plant Edibility Test. Trust me, you'll be expecting to trip, but more than likely, you'll fall.

If you've found a plant with none of the warning signs above, it may be a candidate for the following test.

Universal Plant Edibility Test

Test only one potential food plant at a time.

1. Separate the plant into its basic components:
   a. Leaves
   b. Stems
   c. Roots
   d. Buds
   e. Flowers
2. Smell the food for strong or acid odors. Remember: smell alone does not indicate whether a plant is edible or inedible.
3. Do not eat for eight hours before starting the test.
4. During the eight hours you abstain from eating, test for contact poisoning by placing a piece of the plant part you are testing on the inside of your elbow or wrist. Usually, fifteen minutes is enough time to allow for a reaction.
5. During the test period, take nothing by mouth except purified water and the plant part you are testing.
6. Select a small portion of a single part and prepare it the way you plan to eat it.
7. Before placing the prepared plant part in your mouth, touch a small portion (a pinch) to the outer surface of your lip to test for burning or itching.
8. If, after three minutes, there is no reaction on your lip, place the plant part on your tongue, holding it there for fifteen minutes.
9. If there is no reaction, thoroughly chew a pinch and hold it in your mouth for fifteen minutes. *Do not swallow.*
10. If no burning, itching, numbing, stinging, or other irritation occurs during the fifteen minutes, swallow the food.
11. Wait eight hours. If any ill effects occur during this period, induce vomiting and drink a lot of water.
12. If no ill effects occur, eat one-quarter cup of the same plant prepared the same way. Wait another eight hours. If no ill effects occur, the plant part as prepared is safe for eating.

Remember to test all parts of the plant for edibility, as some plants have both edible and inedible parts. Do not assume that a part that proved edible when cooked is also edible when raw. Test the part raw to ensure edibility before eating it raw. The same part or plant may produce varying reactions in different individuals.

One note about the edibility test: if there is not enough of the plant around to support you, do not waste your time testing it. Don't spend several days testing a plant you will only eat once. Just skip it.

The lists below assume you have prior knowledge of plant edibility or will perform an edibility test.

Examples of Wild Plants With Edible Parts in Different Zones

Temperate Zones

- Amaranth
- Arrowroot
- Beechnut
- Blackberries
- Burdock
- Cattail
- Chestnut
- Chicory
- Chufa
- Dandelion
- Daylily
- Nettle
- Oaks
- Persimmon
- Plantain
- Pokeweed
- Prickly pear cactus
- Purslane
- Sassafras
- Sheep sorrel
- Strawberries

- Thistle
- Water lily and lotus
- Wild onion and garlic
- Wild rose
- Wood sorrel

Tropical Zones

Bamboo

- Bananas
- Breadfruit
- Cashew nuts
- Coconut
- Mango
- Palms
- Papaya
- Sugarcane
- Taro

Desert Zones

Acacia

- Agave
- Cactus
- Date palm
- Desert amaranth

Berries

Green, yellow, or white: 10 percent of varieties are edible.

- Red: 50 percent of varieties are edible.
- Purple, blue, or black: 55 percent of varieties are edible.

- Aggregate berries (thimbleberries, raspberries, blackberries): 99 percent of varieties are edible.

Edible Seaweeds

Dulse

- Green seaweed
- Kelp
- Laver
- *Mojaban*
- Sugar wrack

Pine Trees (Not Just for Teas)

Pine bark is a good source of vitamin C. Scrape away the outer bark, and strip the inner bark. Eat the inner bark raw, dried, cooked, or crushed into flour.

Primal Gathering

Your ancestors would know how to use almost every plant they came across. You do not need their breadth of knowledge to survive. But, at a minimum, you should familiarize yourself with the plant resources that are abundant in your area.

CHAPTER 10

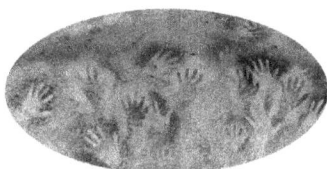

KINESICS: WHAT BODY LANGUAGE IS TELLING YOU

You go to the department store. All around you, people speak to each other, whether they are groups of friends, families with young children, or employees helping customers.

But then, something catches your eye: a young man dressed in ratty clothes snooping about, turning his head as if looking out for something. He is stiff, and he moves with a slow pace. He avoids eye contact with everyone, and he hides from the staff. You think to yourself, *That man is shoplifting.*

Why? Because of his kinesics.

The term *kinesics* was coined in the 1950s by anthropologist Ray Birdwhistell to describe how the head, torso, limbs, and feet communicate messages to others; however, we can expand that idea to include *all* nonverbal communication, such as expressions, gestures, posture, voice, tone, and pitch.

That said, body language is only one part of kinesics; there are also clothing, makeup, and tattoos because what you wear also sends a message. If you dress like a gangbanger, people will react to you in a negative way; if you dress in a suit and tie, you will get a very different reaction. Thus, kinesics can be summed up as what you say with your body and how that body appears to others.

The Four Zones of Nonverbal Communication: Head, Torso, Limbs, Feet

As stated before, the head, the torso, the limbs, and the feet form the basics of kinesics. Of these four, the limbs are the most important because they are not only the source of all gestures but also the weapons of the body; if someone wants to assault you, they will use their hands in some way. Thus, it pays to watch the other person's hands.

For example, if you're in a conversation with someone and they feel uncomfortable, they will cross their arms over their body as if to protect themselves. If they're distracted, they will reach for their phone. If they want to hurt you, they will reach for a gun, or they'll reach for *you*.

But hands can also send specific signals: a thumbs-up shows approval, a middle finger shows anger, a pointing index finger calls attention to something, and raised fists indicate a readiness to fight.

Though hands are important, they are not the only body part that reflects a person's mood. Turning the torso away also indicates discomfort with an interaction; the person wants to move away from the situation but cannot for one reason or another. Pointing the feet and head away shows intent to flee—where are the exits? Is this the right time? Head movement matters because we get most of our information through our eyes and ears.

Consider the emblems that replace words: head nods to indicate yes (up and down) or no (side to side), rubbing the neck or eyes, exhaling a lot, et cetera. These never happen by themselves, but rather alongside other cues in a cluster.

Clusters of Cues

Clusters can be separated into two broad types: behavioral and focus.

Behavioral clusters indicate dominance versus submission or comfort versus discomfort. A dominant person gives off dominant body language—taking up space, leaning in, widening their stance—while a submissive person freezes up or tries to minimize their presence so they don't appear to be a threat. Trying to look harmless is submissive behavior, meant to placate the other party and acknowledge their dominance. Someone comfortable in a situation has relaxed body language; by contrast, someone uncomfortable in a situation tries to pacify themselves by closing their eyes, turning away, rubbing their arms, et cetera because they're squirming under pressure and anticipate some kind of punishment.

Focus clusters show comfort and discomfort through attention to certain things in the environment. That person needs no words; if they want to run away, it'll show. If they think someone is watching, it'll show. If they're afraid of how others will see them, it'll show. If they're *not* afraid, it'll show.

Keep this in mind when deciding what to wear.

Clothing Cues

The idea of "expressing yourself" is popular: say what you want, do what you want, wear what you want, and ignore the norms you're expected to follow. Such expression is meant to show that you're free from the arbitrary restrictions society places on you and that you are not a sheep.

All this expression, however, doesn't account for how everyone will react to you before you open your mouth.

Take clothing, the first thing people notice about you. Wherever you go, there are things considered appropriate to wear or things it's common to wear. Ignoring those norms asks others to pay the cost of trust for you. By showing up in inappropriate clothing, you show that you either do not know the norms or do not respect them. Either way, you become more difficult to trust; no one knows if you are a threat or if you plan to disrupt that environment in other ways. If you are new to a place, this is dangerous because first impressions stick.

If you dress inappropriately on purpose, it is a dominance display: through your clothing, you demand that everyone accept your presence and change the norms to suit you. Displays of dominance create friction, and you cannot be sure that everyone will back down. Even if they don't challenge you in the open, they will be chilly toward you, and it will be difficult to navigate that environment.

By contrast, observing dress norms is a social lubricant, making you easier to trust. Through your clothing, you show that you are reasonable and that you want to cooperate with everyone. Few people will see you as dangerous or disruptive, simplifying communication. The environment will not be as tense, and everyone will be calm. You do not impose any emotional cost on anyone.

That said, "appropriate dress" depends on context. For example, when seeking employment at a craft brewery in Seattle, you would wear a T-shirt, jeans, and piercings to the interview, not a three-piece suit. The opposite is true if you were seeking employment on Wall Street. An anime convention would allow weird costumes; a formal state dinner would not. Know the context of the space you want to enter.

Keep in mind that context can change even if your behavior doesn't. For example, at a nudist retreat, you must be unclothed; showing up dressed is considered indecent. However, if you wander away without clothes on, you will be given strange looks or told to go back to the retreat because now you are the indecent one. Your behavior did not change; only your context did.

And both behavior and context extend beyond clothes.

Behavior in Context

Just as there are appropriate clothes, there are appropriate behaviors, and these, too, depend on what's happening. For example, you expect basketball to be played on a basketball court; you would wonder what was going on if everyone was playing soccer or tennis there instead. Swearing at a bar is different from swearing in church. Shouting at a rock concert is different from shouting in a day care. In any given context, there is an expected baseline of appropriate behavior; much like with clothes, violating these norms is a dominance display and will bring you friction while observing these norms is a show of cooperation and will smooth out your interactions.

The same applies in the other direction as well: from you to the environment. You know something is abnormal when someone behaves in a way inappropriate to that environment, so you pay close attention, then react to any sign of danger. You only have one life, so you can't afford to ignore such signs.

But if someone skulks around a safe place like they fear assassination, you have a cluster mismatch. Abnormal behavior in a given environment *should* demand your attention; you should not be seeing dominance behavior in a coffee shop or fearful behavior at a zoo. As before, pay attention to clusters of behaviors and people; either they may be in danger, or they may be a danger to others. One can determine this by looking at what the person or people are paying attention to.

All this comes back to baselines—what is normal. Not just reading others' signals, but giving off the right ones yourself.

Society at large condemns such behavior as "jumping to conclusions" or "stereotyping," but stereotypes are tested every day, and they survive this testing. Someone sneaking around is up to no good. Someone swaggering up to you with a scowl has ill intent. Someone watching a specific house every day will attempt a break-in.

This is different from a caricature, when you declare someone a threat based on demographics alone. Stereotypes are based on observed actions, while caricatures are based on perceived identities. The more someone's behavior deviates from the norm of a place, the more you should pay attention because that person has demonstrated that they want to impose their will on everyone around them by forcing everyone to pay the cost of trusting them.

Someone who does this with confidence may seem admirable, but because they're willing to defy accepted norms, they may have ill intent.

Observe everyone's reactions; if there's widespread discomfort, you know something's wrong.

But even if a situation isn't dangerous, it pays to watch how everyone interacts. For example, you may see a guy flip another guy off, then the second guy flips him off in return, and they both laugh. This signals that either those guys have a close relationship or such greetings are normal in a place like this.

And once you've observed these behaviors, you should model them to fit in. That said, make sure you understand the context of *all* the interactions because you need to tell the close friends from the complete strangers. Lucky for you, their body language will tell you what you need to know.

The face is less important than you think since it's easy to read a facial expression. If someone's close enough for you to read their face, you've already deemed them safe, or they're already threatening you. The time to spot anomalies is before they get close.

The idea of behavioral kinesics is so embedded in our psyche that it can be summed up simply: "When in Rome, do as the Romans do." Although this can include speech, note the focus on action. Your actions state your truth because you choose those actions. Kinesics covers 60 to 65 percent of our communication, and yet it is not taught in school. Instead, the main focus is on spoken and written language, which, while important, is only a small part of the picture.

Think about why internet discourse is so toxic: all you have is the words, this tiny proportion of our communication arsenal. Most times, you don't even have tone of voice to guide you, making it impossible to spot the kinesic anomalies that would otherwise act as red flags.

On top of all that, most internet discourse takes place on social media, which runs all spaces together and makes it impossible to enforce any kind of localized norm. These mismatched norms set off someone's discomfort cues, then that uncomfortable person seeks allies and gangs up on the threat, leading to the much-feared online mobs. The "anomaly" is purged, but then the cycle repeats.

Kinesic Anomalies to Beware

Your typed words can lie, but your body does not. Many of your bodily motions are automatic, making it hard to hide your intent from those who can spot it. These motions are so hard to control because the limbic system, which handles the fight-or-flight response, causes these motions when you are on edge. Even worse, you are afraid of looking suspicious, making you more nervous and giving off even more tells. This is what police look for when interviewing suspects since the average person cannot control their limbic reactions.

A famous example is former president Bill Clinton's claim that he didn't have an affair with Monica Lewinsky. If you watch a clip of it, you will notice him nodding the whole time; these nods give away the lie. "Actions speak louder that words" is not only about personal responsibility but also about kinesics.

Another common kinesic anomaly is smuggling behavior. When a person gets their gun permit for the first time, they check their bodies to make sure their gun is still there. Likewise, when someone is carrying drugs, they check to make sure they still have their package. That said, it does not even have to be guns or drugs because people do this with their phones all the time, much to the joy of pickpockets, who now know where to look. While smuggling behavior is not threatening on its own, it is something to pay attention to.

Then there is the opposite type of behavior: acting normal. Of course, this is not acting normal, but rather trying to suppress the limbic tells. Since this requires effort, it acts as yet another tell, because the motions will be mechanical.

They will move too fast or too slow. They will move in a precise way. They will look straight ahead and focus only on walking. One can only notice this mechanical behavior when one knows what the person or people normally act like.

Another way mechanical behavior manifests is when someone is doing something or looking at something they should not be, and they want to hide it from you so you don't catch them. They will stiffen up and stare at something. They will focus on their task with an intensity they have never shown before. They will glance at you from the corner of their eye to make sure you do not probe. Yet these behaviors, meant to appear natural, are not so because they are trying to prevent other tells from giving the person's real plans away.

Yet by demonstrating your ability to spot these tells, you could give yourself away. Situational awareness is not normal behavior; looking out for kinesic anomalies makes you look as suspicious as the people you're watching. Observing the crowd, checking the exits, avoiding windows—all these represent anomalies because situational awareness is not done unless under threat. Thus, vigilance can signal fear and, therefore, weakness. In a restaurant, this will not be an issue, but in a bad part of town, it can be costly. Just like you mastered your native tongue, you should master the language of kinesics.

Kinesics Is Communication

Kinesics—nonverbals—is a language all its own, a language that most people don't study. Thus, reading others' kinesics and being mindful of your own put you ahead of the game. When you can identify threats and dangerous situations, you can avoid being murdered or injured, staying well left of bang.

Knowledge of kinesics can help anyone and everyone. For example, if a young black man encounters a group of drunken white men at the local sports bar, and they are chatting and laughing among themselves, he is not in any danger. However, if he encounters those same drunken white men on his way home from work, and they approach him with aggressive intent, the situation has changed, and he must take action.

Note that kinesics varies across cultures; for example, Asian cultures do not value eye contact; South American countries do a lot more touching; and in the Middle East, good male friends often hold hands. Only observation lets you pick up on the norms of a place; even in the locations mentioned here, you have to see what everyone else is doing before you do it, too, lest you send the wrong message.

If you are worried about your new situation, it will show in your discomfort cues. Most people will not confront you; instead, they will do things like move away from you, turn away when you speak to them, and give other signs to show that you are not welcome. By learning the correct signals, you can make yourself at home anywhere.

Further Suggested Reading on Kinesics

Kinesics, unlike straightforward topics like cordage and water purification, has no practical step-by-step tutorials. It's situational; you can only "hear" what someone's body language is saying if you're "listening." And active listening to nonverbals is a skill that requires both study and real-world application.

While the best teacher is experience, here are a few books to help you understand kinesics better so you can read people like a world-class negotiator. After finishing *The Primal Primer*, I suggest you read these:

- For high-stakes communication, *Never Split the Difference* by Chris Voss
- For speed-reading body language, *What Every Body Is Saying* by Joe Navarro
- For building trust with anyone, *How to Win Friends and Influence People* by Dale Carnegie
- For generating small talk, *How to Make People Like You in 90 Seconds or Less* by Nicholas Boothman
- For reading the signals of others, *How to Judge People by What They Look Like* by Edward Dutton

CHAPTER 11

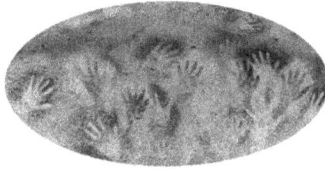

FIRE: SURVIVAL OF THE HOTTEST

How would you fare against a six-year-old in a battle of survival? Do you think you would win? Care to put money on it? I'd take that bet, especially if you were up against my daughter.

My wife and I homeschool our children. Most of the homeschooling happens outdoors. Even in the middle of winter, we're outdoors. It doesn't matter if there's ten feet of snow on the ground. You will find us outside.

Our kids build a fire as part of their educational process first thing each day. They know what kinds and amounts of materials to gather to make the fire. Do you?

My kids also know how to use the fire. They cook lunch on it and use it to boil water and dry out wet clothes. I also get them to ask themselves what else they can use the fire for. We start teaching our kids as soon as possible.

That brings us to my six-year-old daughter. While other kids her age are on tablets, my daughter is stacking logs and setting them ablaze. If society comes crashing down, she'll be able to emerge from the ash and thrive. Will you?

That is why my money is on her. While building a fire isn't essential, it will give you an advantage. It will take time and effort, but when you get a fire going, there's no stopping you.

Read on to learn how to be unstoppable.

Making Fire Made Us Human

How come we're only now talking about fire eleven chapters in? Making a fire combines several of the skills you have already learned throughout this book. So consider this your graduation.

Humans have been around for 6 million years, but we only discovered fire 800,000 years ago. We got along fine without it. You may not ever need to make a fire in a survival situation. But as a tool, it is a force multiplier.

Similar to cordage, fire does not address a specific need. But it does make providing for your needs much easier. That's the main reason it is included as a core human competency.

Making a fire takes patience, practice, perseverance, and most of all preparation. Making fire by hand is hard work, but the energy you put in will be worth it when you see that smoke and hear that crackle. Let's look at the three elements necessary for building a fire.

The Fire Triangle: Oxygen, Fuel, and Heat

The fire triangle consists of the three components that are essential to igniting and sustaining a fire: heat, fuel, and oxygen. If just one of the trinity is removed, the triangle will collapse, and the fire will be extinguished.

Because it's in the air, oxygen is the most readily available component. Controlling the amount of oxygen that reaches your heat source is how you control your fire.

The fuel can be any combination of natural materials that will catch and sustain a flame. Wood is the most common, but you can also use grasses, brush, leaves, cacti, and even animal dung. Whichever fuel you use, the drier the better.

The most challenging part of the fire triangle is generating the heat. That is the skill we need to practice and develop.

Preparing a Fire

Gathering Fuel

When moving through your environment, be on the lookout for materials to make your fire. Find the driest materials you can. If the environment is wet, look for vertical dead plants. Anything lying on the ground will contain moisture, which means you'll have to dry it out first. And that will be a drain on your resources.

Fire requires fuel. Fuels can be broken down into three categories:

- Tinder: the smallest materials, easy to ignite and quick to catch flame.
- Kindling: material as thick as your thumb. It will burn long enough to transfer heat and flame to larger fuel.
- Fuel: the largest material that will sustain the fire for the longest amount of time.

Once you have your material, you'll need to convert it into usable fuel. Much as you can break down bark and stalks into fibers for cordage, you can also use them as tinder. Snap twigs and small branches to create kindling. Break larger branches against trees or rocks to create fuel. Keep an eye out for larger materials already broken down into adequate sizes.

How much material will you need? A good practice is to collect enough material to make three fires before beginning your first. This allows you to move up or down the fire-making steps as needed. Fire making takes practice, so you must be ready to try, try, again.

A note about wetness: if you're in an environment with heavy rainfall, then much of the wood you collect will be damp. Stack the wood from driest to wettest with the driest at the bottom and wettest at the top. Keep in mind that vertical dead trees will be drier than horizontal living branches.

Remember, our ancestors had the worst living situation we could imagine. No electricity. No running water. No temperature control. Average humans today die of exposure if lost in the wilderness for several days.

Don't let that happen to you. Choose the right site to build your fire. Here's how . . .

Site Selection

Select a flat, level site. Clear away as much existing material as possible. Your aim is to get down to the raw earth. If the ground is wet or covered in snow, line rocks or sticks next to each other to create a platform to build your fire on. Layer as many levels as you need to get your fire off the wet surface. Build your fire as close to your shelter as possible. But not too close! You want the fire to warm you for the rest of the night, not the rest of your life.

The Bird's Nest

Next, use the kindling to form a loose ball or "bird's nest" the size of your fist. As you crunch the larger pieces together, smaller bits will fall off. Create the bird's nest from the larger pieces, then press your thumb into the ball to create a shallow divot. Collect the kindling that fell away, and place it into the divot. This will be where you place the ember or coal you'll generate later.

You will need to make quick transitions at each part of the fire-making process. With your tinder prepared, arrange your kindling and fuel near the site you've cleared for your fire.

If you are working in wet conditions, you may need to scrape the damp exterior off your materials. You will also need to add kindling and fuel to your fire more slowly. This will allow the existing heat to dry the materials as they're added without putting out the fire.

Stack and Flow

When you first generate an ember or coal, gently blow on it to increase the heat output. Keep blowing on it when you add it to your tinder until the tinder ignites. From there, you will either add your tinder to the kindling or add the kindling to your tinder.

After that, you'll add the fuel. There are two ways to arrange it:

Teepee Stack Method

The teepee stack forms as you lay fuel on your ignited kindling. Prop your fuel onto your kindling. Work your way around in a circle. Keep one end on the surface and the other forming an apex above your flame. This structure provides good light and heat. But keep in mind it will burn fast as oxygen can reach all parts of the fire. If you use this method, you will need to add fuel continuously.

Parallel Log Method

Begin the same way as the teepee method. But as you add fuel material, lay it parallel to the wind and lay each piece of material parallel to the others. This will look like the log stack in a lumber yard. This method limits the airflow, reducing the flame size. And as the fuel burns down, it will create a bed of hot coals rather than big bright flames. These coals are ideal for cooking on.

Generating Heat: Friction

Most primitive and ancestral approaches to fire rely on friction to generate heat. The two most common ways of making a primitive fire are the hand drill and the bow drill.

The Hand Drill or "Rubbing Two Sticks Together"

To make a hand drill fire, you need a hearth board or fireboard and a spindle that spins inside it. These pieces need to be bone dry.

Spindle

The spindle must be straight and a bit soft. Quick-growing plants with straight stalks like cattail, horseweed, and goldenrod work well, but any straight piece of sturdy woody material can be used.

- Find straight material roughly one-half inch in diameter.
- Cut or break the material into eighteen-inch lengths: the distance from your elbow to your fingertip.
- Scrape off any knobs or thorns, and make the spindle smooth. This will help save your hands from going raw later.
- Scrape or cut the larger end to fit inside the notch of the hearth board.
- Remove any frayed pieces from the end. These will disrupt the dust pile the friction is creating.
- Once you've prepared your spindle, do not put it on the ground; place it somewhere dry.

Hearth Board/Fireboard

The hearth board must be made out of nonresinous wood. That means no conifer trees. It also needs to be made from soft wood. Press your fingernail into the wood. Does it leave a dent? If it does, you're using the right material.

- Find a material you can split into pieces one-half to three-quarters of an inch thick.
- Cut or break the material into twelve-inch to eighteen-inch lengths.
- Split the material vertically to create a flat surface to work on.

- Using a sharp tool, a rock, or harder piece of wood, create a divot near one edge. This is where you'll place the spindle.
- Slowly spin the spindle in the divot, applying downward force. This will deepen the divot and seat the spindle.
- Cut a notch along the side of the hearth board that breaks the divot's wall to funnel all the dust created by friction.
- The divot with the notch should look like a pizza with a slice missing.

Using the Hand Drill

Place the hearth board on the tinder or a piece of bark you'll use to collect and transfer the ember or coal to the tinder.

- Hold the hearth board down with your foot.
- Place the spindle into the hearth board divot.
- Hold the top of the spindle between your hands.
- Rapidly spin the spindle between your hands, sliding your palms against each other from wrist to fingertip and back again. Keep applying downward force.
- When you reach the bottom of the spindle, return your hand to the top and begin spinning the spindle again with a quick, fluid motion.
- Use speed, not force. Start slow if needed and pick up the pace as you get comfortable with the movement.
- Smoke will appear as the friction creates wood dust and the heat from the friction begins to ignite it.
- The dust will collect in the notch, and you will see it turn from brown to black as it begins to char.
- Continue to spin until you can see a hot red ember in the char or until the char smokes even when you stop spinning.
- Carefully transfer the lit char into the prepared tinder ball.
- Gently blow on the tinder ball to help the ember ignite the tinder.
- Once at least half the tinder is aflame, place the tinder ball into your fire pit and begin to add kindling.

- Continue to gently blow on the tinder and kindling until the kindling has ignited.
- Add more kindling until the kindling will sustain the flames.
- Begin to add fuel material to sustain the fire.

The Bow Drill or "Spin It"

Making a bow drill fire requires five elements. Like the hand drill, you'll need a hearth board or fireboard and a spindle. You'll also need a bearing block to hold the spindle in place and a piece of bent wood to use as the bow. You'll also need some cordage for the bowstring.

Bearing Block

The bearing block holds the spindle in place as the bowstring rotates the spindle. You can use a piece of harder wood that you can carve a divot into. Or use a shell or rock with a natural indentation that will function as a divot.

Bow and Bowstring

Collect a curved piece of wood to use as a bow. Use cordage to make a bowstring, tying it to either end of the bow with a little slack to allow for the spindle.

Using the Bow Drill

The bow drill operates in a similar manner to the hand drill. It is used as follows:

- Place the hearth board directly on the tinder or a piece of bark you will use to collect and transfer the ember or coal to the tinder.
- Hold the hearth board down with your weak foot (i.e., your left foot if you're right handed).

- Insert the spindle between the bow and the bowstring. Twist the bowstring to loop it around the spindle.
- Place the spindle into the hearth board divot.
- Hold the bearing block with your weak hand.
- Brace your weak arm against the leg holding the hearth board in place.
- Seat the top of the spindle into the bearing block divot. Press down firmly.
- With your strong hand, slide the bow back and forth to spin the spindle rapidly.
- Use speed, not force. Start slower if you need to, and pick up speed as you get comfortable with these movements.
- Smoke will appear as friction creates and starts to ignite wood dust.
- The dust will collect in the notch, and you will see it turn from brown to black as it begins to char.
- Continue to spin until you can see a hot red ember in the char or until the char smokes even when you stop spinning.
- Carefully transfer the lit char into the prepared tinder ball.
- Gently blow on the tinder ball to help the ember ignite the tinder.
- Once at least half the tinder is aflame, place the tinder ball into your fire pit and begin to add kindling.
- Continue to gently blow on the tinder and kindling until the kindling has ignited.
- Add more kindling until the kindling will sustain the flames.
- Begin to add fuel material to sustain the fire.

Bonus: The Dakota Fire Pit or "Stealth Fires"

The Dakota fire pit is a high-heat, low-smoke fire. It uses less fuel than a standard fire because the fire is below ground level controlling for airflow, which makes it harder for others to see the flames.

Here's how to build it:

- Dig an eight- to twelve-inch diameter hole eighteen to twenty-four inches deep.
- Then dig a second, smaller hole to the same depth twelve to eighteen inches upwind of the first.
- Connect the bottoms of the two holes.
- Load the larger hole with kindling and fuel.
- Light a tinder ball and add it to the kindling to start the fire.
- Place stones or green sticks across the top of the fire pit to use for cooking.

Nothing without Fire

Modern humans would not exist without fire. Fire allowed for more calorie consumption every day from foods gathered and hunted in nature. Fire making is *the* essential modern skill. Nothing gives you a more immediate sense of control over yourself and your environment than making fire.

The truth is we're *all* in a survival situation twenty-four seven. It's easy to forget because we're surrounded by conveniences that hide that reality from us. Your water heater needs fire. Your car needs fire. The power company needs fire. If you're not making fire, you're dependent on other people who do, all day every day.

Imagine that the most incompetent politician on earth is responsible for you and your family's survival. If that doesn't terrify you, you're not going to make it.

But it's not like I'm against tools like matches. If you have access to dry matches and you're stuck out in the wilderness, use them. At the same time, you must still be able to make fire without matches.

It's not about always playing on hard mode. It's about survival. Use any available leverage to ensure that you survive. The best advantage you can give yourself is reassuring your brain that you can survive without man-made resources. Being unstoppable means being able to walk naked into the woods and build a fire. Just like your ancestors did.

Laws, ethics, and codes can vary across time and place. But fire is a constant. It provides heat. It provides light. It provides life. Get practicing.

CHAPTER 12

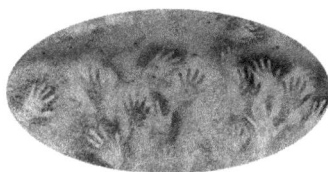

BIOMETRICS:
HOW YOUR BODY TRIES
TO SAVE YOUR LIFE

How can you keep it together when you're a nervous wreck? When it comes down to it, will you sail true, or are you going to run aground? While you think about those questions, let me tell you a story.

Mean Man with a Short Temper

When my training partner Larry wasn't angry at me in the four-by-four ring, he was busy being angry at everyone else. Sometimes you just had to make sure you were out of his way.

That guy was a ball of rage, and the military was the best place for him. One time, I asked him what he'd be doing if he wasn't in the marines. He smiled and said, "Time."

I let him finish playing five-finger filet in peace after that.

Seeing Larry train made me glad he was on our side. Even without an M16, he was dangerous. A stone mountain with the reach of an orangutan, his mind was as tough as his body. This guy was scary.

Even if you did whatever you could to not piss him off, Larry's fuse could be lit with a glance. The drill instructors tried to channel that anger into something more constructive. It seemed like nothing could break him. But they were sure there had to be something that could bring him back down to ground level.

Slide for Life

One of the exercises we had to complete in marine boot camp was the slide for life. We had to climb up a hundred-foot tower and down a rope with a transition to hand over hand at the halfway point.

It was a bit of a thrill watching our fellow recruits complete the exercise. And even though a fierce competitive streak ran through our group, we supported each other. We went up in twos. Guess who I got paired with?

Larry and I made the hundred-foot climb. The wind cut through us like a knife. At the same time, I realized that as soon as we left the platform, the hard part would be over.

I don't like heights much, but I still could talk myself into going over the edge of the platform. Everything was quiet, but then the smell hit me. At first, I thought it was coming from the bay or the nearby airfield or something. Either way, it smelled bad, and I said to my buddy, "Got to love that ocean air!"

He did not respond.

The closer I got to him, the worse the smell got. I asked him if he was all right. Dead air.

Panic crept in. He was sheet white and smelled of sheets, too—not the fresh kind, though.

I always thought "I crapped my pants with fear" was just a figure of speech. It turned out to be based in reality. With a laugh, I told my buddy to snap out of it. But he was staring at the ground in a trance, his mouth contorting in silent prayer.

What was I supposed to do? There was a chance he was going to take the world's messiest shortcut. I wanted to reach out and grab him, but I knew there was a good chance that doing so could make things worse.

He Had to Reason

I signaled for the drill instructor. He joined us on the rope, and I told him what was happening.

The drill instructor observed the situation, then unleashed a torrent of verbal abuse on Larry so strong it threatened to sweep me away, too.

It took him a moment, but my buddy returned to the land of the conscious. The color returned to his face. I realized that fear had taken over his body, and only now was he back in control.

He was lucky it happened in a safe environment. Had that been an active war zone, his odds of making it down in one piece would have been cut drastically.

But in the end, he descended. Larry never got over his fear of heights, though.

It Can Happen to You

You might be wondering why I told that story. Let it sink in that the scariest guy in our platoon lost his mystique the second he got six feet off the ground. The joke was "How do you stop yourself from getting whupped by Larry? Climb."

Larry's body turned on him. If it can happen to the meanest marine, then imagine what can happen to you.

While you never know when your body might betray you, one thing you can do is plan for it. Let's take a look at how.

Why Now?

Let's look at everything you are now in control of. You can find shelter and control your environment. You can forage to stave off starvation. You can make fires to control your heat level and prevent death from exposure.

This is the first topic in this book that you have no control over. We've covered environmental baselines, spotting anomalies in those baselines, and considering proxemics to find an anomaly's source. Kinesics tells you what needs your attention. Is someone shivering or fidgeting when they shouldn't?

Biometrics is the last link in the chain. It takes you from your external environment and into your body, which is always talking to you. Can you understand what it's saying? Getting it right could mean the difference between life and death.

In the story above, my training buddy's body yelled at him, "You're gonna fall! You're gonna die!" That voice shouted so loud, it disabled his ability to think. Instinct took over. He was in a harness. Unless he cut it, there was no way he could have come to harm. It did not matter to him. All his body saw was a long fall.

Look at the people around you. Is anyone beet red or ghostly pale? Red means anger, and pale means fear. Keeping that in mind will help you predict outcomes. It will not guarantee optimal outcomes, but you will be in a better position to avoid being taken unaware.

Knowing biometrics could save your life. Think about a mass shooting situation, for instance. Reading the shooter's biometrics might not have saved everyone, but it might have given them more of a chance.

And the power of biometrics can help make you more successful. The best athletes learn biometrics.

Watch a professional golfer's body language. He grips the club and has solid posture with a slight bend in his knees. The golfer raises the club, waits for a moment, then swings. The ball flies high through the air to make a rapid, arcing descent onto the green. Showing no outward reaction, the golfer only surveys the scene and prepares for the next shot.

He takes it, and the ball goes in the hole. The only sign of emotion is a slight fist pump.

Pro golfers are masters of their biometrics. If they let animal instinct kick in, they jeopardize their game. The same goes for poker players. They hold, fold, or ante up based on the other players' biometrics. Dilating pupils or fingers drumming on the table indicate a nervous reaction to the hand dealt. At the same time, they don't want to let anything slip. A twitch of the lip might be the only signal to bust out or go all in.

That's why it was good that my buddy had his moment in training rather than on the battlefield. The military wants you to be a skilled and practiced combatant. Imagine you're deployed to a conflict. You are hunkered behind a wall waiting for reinforcements. There have been sporadic firefights, and you're running low on ammo. All of a sudden, you hear boots on the ground and shouts in your own language. The cavalry has arrived! All they have left to do is scale the wall to get to you.

From the other side, you hear, "I can't climb that! They're on their own."

Military training breaks down all the bad habits picked up over the years and builds up a new system to depend on in a crisis. The marines train your body to free up your mind's creativity. If you need to take out an enemy gun emplacement, your focus needs to be on that, not on whether you can cross the distance without being spotted.

Another example is my friend, ghostwriter Joshua Lisec. He had been chosen to give a TEDx Talk back in 2017. Now, public speaking ranks high among people's fears. Joshua did not want to leave anything to chance on the big day when the lights came on and the cameras rolled, so he implemented an unusual training regime. If you don't know Joshua, you might not know that he lives near a swamp in forested southwest Ohio. Every evening for two months before the TEDx event, he would run through the swamp and recite his speech in the muggy air. *Run*. Not walk.

Over those two months, he adapted to that environment—reciting his speech from memory with a racing heart, pounding pulse, and sweaty palms. And he was able to give his speech with perfect precision; his biometrics were used to adverse conditions. The air-conditioned hall where the TEDx Talk took place felt like paradise after the murky swamp, Joshua told me.

Biometric awareness can make or break a career. It has the power to save or end a life. That may sound extreme, but with incidents of violence on the rise, ask yourself if it's a risk you want to take.

What Is Biometrics?

We've mentioned biometrics throughout this chapter already, and I still owe you a proper definition. Here we go.

Biometrics is the observation, measurement, and calculation of our physiological response to stress, fear, and threats: in essence, any external stimuli. Biometric cues are tied to our physiological and psychological needs. When our needs are being met, our bodies maintain their normal state of equilibrium. When our bodies register a change in the environment, they will adapt to the new conditions.

Your midbrain controls your limbic system. This cues your automatic responses to changes triggered by hormones your body releases. When the environmental baseline changes, your body adapts. When an anomaly is introduced, the body responds to this new stressor. And your fight, flight, and freeze response provides new cues.

Midbrain

Your midbrain comprises several systems working in conjunction. They are:

- Limbic system
- Autonomic nervous system
- Sympathetic/parasympathetic
- Emotion, reflex, and survival response
- The five *F*s (the root of Maslow's hierarchy of needs)
  - Food
  - Fornication
  - Fight

- Flight
- Freeze

Chemical Brain Dump

Adrenaline (prepare for action)

- Cortisol (protect the body)
- Dopamine (keep us going)

Getting a feeling that something is off doesn't mean you're paranoid. That feeling, whether you call it butterflies in your stomach or a gut instinct, evolved over millions of years to alert you of subtle changes in your environment. When your limbic system tells you there's an anomaly in the area, it's up to you to determine if your gut is in line with reality.

This is why it's important to be in control of your biometrics. You've got to interpret those cues in context. Some of these responses are uncontrollable. Think of listening to your body like dealing with a baby or a dog. You know it's trying to tell you something, but it can't come right out and tell you. Search for clues. You must be a detective in your environment.

As important as it is to read yourself, you must also be able to read the people around you. Learn to pick up the signals others are sending about their emotional and physical states. When you have done that, you can identify the baseline, and from there, you can establish anomalies and infer intent.

One of the most recognizable universal responses is the flinch. We raise our hands to protect our brains when startled or threatened suddenly.

Let's look at some more cues to pick up on.

Common Biometric Cues

- Tunnel vision
  - Loss of peripheral vision and restriction of focus
- Facial and extremity flushing (vasodilation—anger/shame)
- Facial and extremity paling (vasoconstriction—fear/stress)

- Dry mouth
- Pupil dilation (for good things)
- Pupil constriction (for bad things)
- Rapid breathing
- Shaking
- Shivering
- Tremors
- Fidgeting
- Goose bumps
- Muscle tension
- Increased blink rate
- Loss of fine motor control

Emotional Cues

- Anger/Frustration
- Red face
- Flared nostrils
- Increase in breathing rate
- Muscle tension
- Shaking

Fear/Anxiety

- Paling or ashen-looking face
- Shallow/quick breathing
- Increased sweating
- Tremors/shivering
- Goose bumps
- Dry mouth

Contempt/Disgust

- Increased breathing
- Increased salivation/swallowing

Does It Fit?

When evaluating biometric cues, ask yourself, *Does the cue fit the situation?* That's how you spot anomalies. Shivering results from the body diverting blood flow from the extremities to the major internal organs. It may occur when someone is anxious, afraid, or angry. Or just cold.

Each situational awareness tool must be used in conjunction with the others to discern whether a given cue is a change in your baseline or an anomaly. And another cue category to watch for is the parasympathetic responses to the hormone dump.

Parasympathetic Backlash

Adrenaline, the "fight, flight, or freeze" hormone, can have the reverse effect, slowing heart rate and breathing to restore equilibrium. This can lead to observable cues such as sleepiness, yawning, lethargy, and disorientation.

Think back to the story from Chapter 4. My wife and my friend were oblivious to the men tailing us. I couldn't even tell you what they looked like because I was focused on having a good time. The moment I detected a threat, tunnel vision kicked in. I missed all their biometric cues, and my own took over.

My size and military training were my only advantages over our assailants. What if I'd been smaller and had no military training?

Learning biometric cues is more likely to save you from danger than martial arts or firearms training. Even law enforcement officers can fall prey to their own biometrics. I suspect this is what happened during the tragic Uvalde, Texas, elementary school shooting, when armed law enforcement officers could not bring themselves to enter the building. Children were murdered by a lone gunman while a police force stood outside.

You think you'll be the hero until your body won't let you. In some cases, you may not get another chance. Reading about what happened tomorrow is always the best outcome for you and those you love in a bad situation.

CHAPTER 13

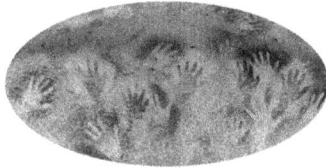

HYGIENE: THE BUSINESS OF DOING YOUR BUSINESS

Have you ever had a culture clash so violent you felt your head spin? While I was in the service, I lived in Japan for just over a year. Some of my friends were already there when I arrived. They threw me a welcoming party. Eating a bunch of food I'd never eaten before and drinking a bunch of drinks I'd never drunk before was a whole new experience for me. And Tokyo was a good place to start.

As the night went on, empty sake bottles piled up. Remnants of rice and sockeye salmon lined our soy sauce trays. Back out in the street, one of my friends suggested karaoke when I felt a rumbling in my stomach. I'd been eating and drinking for a few hours and had put off nature's call as long as I could. Excusing myself, I made my way across the street to a private restroom. How much different could it be?

A lot different, as it turned out.

It was like all of Japan had gotten together to play a joke on me. I didn't see a commode—just a hole in the ground. Had I gone into the wrong stall? Maybe this was the handicapped commode?

To be honest, I was in denial. The hole in the ground was as close as I would get to a toilet. It was a culture shock. At first, I feared I would spend the rest of my time in Japan constipated. But I'd hunted my own food, survived blizzards, and built shelters in the woods. I was not going to let a Japanese bathroom defeat me.

There were no instructions. But there were bars on the sides of the stall. So there I was, three sheets to the wind, pants around my ankles, squatted down hanging onto the bars. I leaned way back so as not to splash myself. My knuckles were whiter than they'd been on roller-coaster rides.

It was horrible, but I learned how to do it right after a few attempts. The experience taught me how Westerners take our hygiene practices for granted.

> Also you shall have a place outside the camp, where you may go out; and you shall have an implement among your equipment, and when you sit down outside, you shall dig with it and turn and cover your refuse.
>
> Deuteronomy 23:12–13
> The New King James Version (NKJV)

Hygiene is important. Even the Good Book has verses dedicated to what to do with your poop. Think about that for a moment. A book with origins stretching back thousands of years wants you to give serious consideration to where you have a bathroom break.

What's interesting is that for 99 percent of human history, the common method of going to the bathroom was closer to how it's done in Japan. In the West, we complicate the process with extra steps. Squatting down is better for your health. It straightens out your colon and takes pressure off your back. Modern toilets may be fashionable, but squatting is a longer tradition. Only now are we beginning to remember this fact, which could explain the popularity of products like the Squatty Potty.

Using toilet paper to clean is another complication. The river used to carry away the waste, and it was nature's bidet, provided you used it downstream from where you drank.

We'll come back to refuse later in this chapter. For now, let's consider the end of the process. After you've done your business, how do you get clean when antibacterial soap from a squirt bottle is unavailable? Hygiene in the wilderness is about more than making sure not to wipe your butt with poison ivy. It's about managing everyday contact with germs, before and after you eat.

Nature finds a way. To learn it, read on.

Tannins

Tannins are bitter and astringent chemical compounds that belong to a larger polyphenols group. They occur abundantly in the bark of many trees and in various leaves, legumes, and fruits. Tannins protect against insects, bacteria, fungi, and viruses. Their antiseptic, antifungal, antibacterial, and antiviral properties make tannins useful for hygiene purposes.

Common Tannin Plants

All plants contain tannins. They are what give unripe fruit that bitter taste. Plants use tannins to discourage animals and parasites from consuming them. Hardwood trees are high in tannins.

Some plants with high tannin concentrations are:

- Oak: bark, leaves, fruit, galls
- Hickory: bark, leaves, fruit, galls
- Chestnut: bark, leaves, fruit, galls
- Ash: bark, leaves, fruit, galls
- Witch hazel: bark, leaves, fruit, galls

Now that you know where to find them, here's how to use them.

Extracting Tannins: Tannin Tea

Cut live branches from a tree, and shave the bark into a container suitable for boiling water, such as with the hot rock method. Add leaves, and if the tree produces a gall (an abnormal growth), chop it up and add that as well. Add water, then boil the tea and allow it to steep. The water will turn brown. The darker it gets, the higher the tannin concentration.

Tannin tea can be used to clean and disinfect tools, clothes, and your body. It can also be used as a mouthwash. You can mix tannin tea with saponins to create an antibacterial soap, too. Speaking of which . . .

Saponins

Saponins are bitter, plant-derived organic glycosides that foam when agitated in water. They are water and fat soluble, which makes them useful to clean oils from our bodies, like soap.

Common Saponin Plants

Saponins are another plant defense. Many plants produce saponins, but some of the more common are:

- Horse chestnut: nuts (you can even order these on Etsy.com)
- Soapwort: whole plant, especially the roots
- English ivy: leaves
- Soap nut or soapberry tree: berries
- Clematis: leaves and flowers
- Buffalo berry: berries
- Soopolallie: berries
- California soaproot: bulb, roots
- Soapbush tree: leaves
- Soapweed yucca: roots
- Sugar beet: leaves
- Licorice: roots

Extracting Saponin

Fill a container with water. Crush the saponin-containing plant parts, and add the pulp to the water. Agitate the water until a lather forms.

You can extract some saponin directly from parts such as berries. Crush them in your hands, and rub the material over your skin with vigor. Watch as you build up a lather.

Soap

If you don't know what soap is, your family and loved ones will thank you for paying attention to this chapter. Anyway, soap is a substance that can mix with oil and water that's used for cleaning.

Field Soap

To make field soap you will need:

- Container for soaking (burn bowl)
- Container for melting and mixing (burn bowl)
- Tool for mixing (branches)
- Clean water
- Rendered animal fat
- Wood ash
- Cloth for straining
- Mold for soap (burn bowl, shell, cloth, etc.)

To make the soap:

- Soak wood ash in water for twenty-four hours. This will produce lye water. Lye is caustic. Take care during the rest of the preparation. Do not swallow the lye water, and avoid contact with skin and eyes.
- Strain the water mixture into another container and discard the wood ash.

- Melt the rendered fat into a liquid.
- Add the lye water to the liquid fat (two ounces lye water per pound of fat).
- Mix thoroughly to incorporate the lye water fully into the fat.
- Pour the mixture into molds. (Use your straining cloth in your first container, then tie it into a bundle if you have no other mold.)
- Let the molded mixture sit as long as you can. The soap will become less harsh the longer it sits.

Additional Hygiene Materials

Crushed Charcoal

Not always, but often, fire will give you charcoal, which is black, unlike ash, the white stuff. Get charcoal from the fire you learned to make, and grind it up as fine as you can to . . .

- Make mouthwash
- Make toothpaste
- Rub onto skin as antibacterial deodorant

Smoke

Most people think showering with soap is the best way to get clean. But it's not the only way. You can take a "smoke bath" by standing in the smoke of your fire for four to five minutes. It will kill bacteria and reduce odors.

Get into the spread-eagle position. You can stand there with your clothes on, but au naturel is better. Get the fumes into all your cracks and crevices. Take care not to inhale too much smoke.

Direct Sunlight

Ultraviolet light kills bacteria. When you're letting your clothes dry, that's the perfect time for some naked sunbathing. Get some vitamin D. If there are other people with you, you might want to go somewhere else or at least give them a heads up.

Toothbrush

Find a softwood tree or bush, and remove a small branch. Willow is ideal. Pound or crush the end to separate the fibers. Chew the same end to separate them further.

Scrape your teeth from the gumline outward with the fibrous end of the stick. Use another stick that branches in two, processed the same way, to get the backs of your teeth. Grind up some charcoal as fine as you can to reduce abrasion, and make a paste from it to use while brushing. Follow up with tannin tea. Add some mint if you can find any.

Wild Leeks and Onions

These plants make fair insect repellent when you rub them all over your body, though they will repel people as well. You can find leeks and onions in prairies and former corn or soybean fields. Grab a few handfuls and squeeze until you see oils. Spread the oil all over your skin since that's where the odor comes from.

Eats, Poops, and Leaves

Now we're at the main attraction of this chapter. Everything that drinks, pees. Everything that eats, poops.

Establishing good processes for managing your waste is important. Your health depends on developing a robust waste management system. If you don't, you'll get sick. If you get sick, you'll get set back. Your sickness will have a domino effect on every other thing you're trying to do to stay alive. Don't disadvantage yourself.

Where to Go

First things first. Set up an area away from camp to get rid of your waste. It should be at least a couple of hundred feet distant. Make sure your waste is not between you and your water supply. Select a spot downhill and downwind if possible.

Urine

Pee when you feel like you need to. Holding it creates an environment that allows bacteria to grow with ease. It also slows down your body's process of waste removal. This means you won't feel the urge to drink water, even if you need to.

Ladies, use an absorbent material (natural, like moss, or a reusable, cleanable cloth) to wipe. Place a cotton pad in tannin tea overnight. The cotton-like material of a cattail can be used if cotton is unavailable. Lacking even that, use a clean, smooth stick to tap moisture off the area. Then air dry for a couple of minutes.

Feces

When a river is unavailable, use land.

For each use, dig a hole about six inches in diameter and twelve inches deep. Squat over the hole, and deposit your waste. Wipe off with one of the materials discussed below, and discard it into the hole, too. If you can, add some wood ash or charcoal to the hole. This reduces the smell and will prevent attracting attention from insects, rodents, or any larger predators. Cover the hole with the dirt you dug up.

For longer stays with more people, you may need to dig a trench instead of a hole. You can also make going more convenient by adding logs around the hole or trench for support. All the other steps in the process above apply to trenches. Be creative, but be careful.

Always clean up after you go. It is a good idea to have some tannin tea ready to ensure you do not bring any unwanted substances back to camp with you.

What to Wipe With

Your goal here is to create a barrier between your hand and your waste. At the same time, you don't want to use anything that will scratch or irritate your skin. Some materials you can use are:

- Fresh or dry leaves (use layers to avoid breakthroughs)
- Smooth sticks to scrape off waste
- Smooth rocks to scrape off waste
- Moss
- Water to rinse off
- Reusable and washable cloths

The odds you'll ever be in this situation are low. At the same time, they're not zero. You need to know that you can take care of yourself. Every animal has found a way to clean and preen itself. Cleanliness is more than a survival skill; it's an animal instinct that humans think we're too good for. We've become more aware of what goes in our mouths as we've gotten more prudish about the other end. Convenience has killed our connection with nature.

Which makes us more vulnerable to . . .

Other Dangers

If you're in a situation where your life depends on these skills, you learn how weak and compromised you can become in a short time. If you get ill, you will not be able to focus on the threats around you. If you get an infection, there's a chance it could spread to other parts of your body, and you'll die. If you take good care of your hygiene and respond quickly to potential infections, you can take on the bigger challenges you will face.

You are one vacation away from needing these skills, whether for you or someone you come across. Let's look at some of the most common threats.

Whether it's a senior citizen recovering at home from hip replacement surgery or a young adult out on a walk, falling is one of the biggest killers. Twelve thousand people die from falling down the stairs in the United States alone. This is why martial arts trainers teach you how to fall first. Most of us who have access to phones with emergency services nearby should be fine. But what about a worst-case scenario?

Because a serious fall is only ever a few inches away, even on Metropark trails a few miles outside major cities.

Think of surviving in the wilderness like a video game. Your character has one hundred health points. Many things can sap your points away. If you're hungry, you lose ten points; if you're hungry, you can't focus, which means you end up tripping and getting a splinter. That costs you another ten points. The splinter gets infected. Minus another ten. The infection makes you sick. Scratch off another ten.

You get to the point where you're so weak, the wolf that's been hanging about sees a moment and takes it. Mr. Wolf drags you back to his den. You bleed out on the way, but it doesn't matter because you were last in a fever dream about cantaloupe and mimosas.

Do you get the point yet?

Infection and illness may not kill you outright, unless you have a wound that goes gangrenous. But they have a compound effect and will put you in a weakened state. Do you want to suffer a bout of diarrhea while dealing with a broken femur?

I understand that talking about wiping your butt is not as sexy as making fire and hunting for food. Yet it might be one of the most important aspects of sustaining your own survival. Think of this as the prime directive of *The Primal Primer*: always be hygienic.

CHAPTER 14

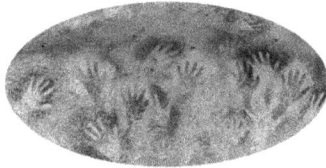

SITUATIONAL AWARENESS: IF SOMETHING FEELS WRONG, IT PROBABLY IS

How can we tell when things are about to go wrong? Is there some-thing inside us that helps us in times of need? If so, can it be trained?

Minnesota has a massive state fair. It lasts a couple of weeks and frequently receives more than 100,000 visitors a day. Families come from all around to enjoy it. My family loves it.

It would be easy to lose one of the kids in such a huge crowd. The last thing we want is to get back to the car and ask, "Didn't we have more kids than this?"

I don't want to take any chances. I want to get everyone home safe, without incident. So my wife and I are vigilant with our children and make sure they never wander too far.

The fair is a great place to practice situational awareness. Where are people in relation to one another? How can I implement proxemics to make sure my kids are safe? Does someone not quite fit in?

It's also easy to notice a change in the atmosphere at the fair. You hear the sound of beer bottles clinking; you taste the cigarette smoke in the air. Groups of young men talk a little louder with each sentence uttered.

It can be tempting to switch off your brain to just enjoy time with the family. But it doesn't hurt to be aware of your surroundings. After all, everything can go south in an instant. And the more you use situational awareness, the more it becomes a habit. In time, it becomes second nature.

Realize that not everyone is as kind and conscientious as you. In fact, some people just don't know how to behave in public. At night in particular. When the moon comes out, you need to be extra cautious. All it takes is one wrong look or an accidental shoulder check for violence to break out. You don't want to be there when it does, much less have your family there.

This is why it's vital to practice situational awareness wherever and whenever you can. That's why it's important to have a cutoff time at outdoor events. Otherwise, you could be putting yourself and your loved ones in a threatening situation.

Maybe you feel confident in the abilities you've developed from *The Primal Primer*. But the point is not to take on groups of rowdy drunks. The point is to assess the situation and get the heck out of there. Listen to your intuition when it says to get out.

If Something Feels Wrong, It Probably Is

We've covered a lot of situational awareness material. The goal is to empower yourself and speed up your decision-making process when confronted with threats.

You've heard people talk about their "gut feelings," and I bet you've been told to "go with your gut" before. *Gut* refers to the limbic system, which has evolved to pick up threatening signals from your environment. Our daily habits inhibit these innate abilities.

When you develop situational awareness, you're supporting your limbic system with skills that adapt it to our ever-changing "civilized" environment. It's no longer enough to trust your gut.

You have to train it, too.

Speeding Up Decision-Making

We observe patterns of behavior on an animal level. Then our rational brains build entire social structures around those habits. We are creatures of habit. We create observable patterns of behavior. No behavior is completely random. We have physiological and biological needs that must be met, and our hardwired behaviors reflect this fact.

Instead of being passive, we can be active and watch how these patterns of behavior unfold to give a proper response. To maximize your chances, you must adopt a hunter's mindset and become a threat profiler. Seek out the patterns that indicate a threat is likely to appear. From there, make a decision about how to handle the situation in advance. Supercharge your decision-making by:

- Being active in searching and observing your environment for these patterns.
- Holding yourself in a state of readiness with an understanding you may need to take action fast.
- Making reasonable, adaptable inferences about the cues you are picking up.

If you're not prepared to make a decision before you spot trouble, trouble will find you. Hesitation could mean death. So don't aim for the perfect response.

Imperfect Decisions

There is no such thing as the perfect decision. No matter how much information you have, you will not have it all. If you wait for all the information, you leave yourself vulnerable to analysis paralysis. And that makes you much more likely to act too late.

A 70 percent–informed decision that leads to immediate action produces better outcomes in threat situations than waiting to be 100 percent informed.

How do you know what 70 percent is and which decision is right? The answer is heuristics.

Heuristic Decision-Making

Heuristics is an approach to decision-making with minimal time and information using practical methods. It also leverages your evolved abilities and the environmental context to determine reasonable—not optimal—short-term action.

Baseline + Anomaly = Decision

The above methods for assessing environments and the people in them for cues also let us use heuristic decision-making. The idea is to assess threat potentials.

As we've stated throughout this material, we are looking for anomalies. And we're using context and relevance to determine if those anomalies warrant action. The more prepared we are for this process, the more likely it is to be successful.

Once we have determined an anomaly exists, how do we use that awareness to make decisions?

Threat Decision Tree
Fight/Flight/Focus

Does the anomaly represent a hostile act, hostile intent, or immediate threat?

If yes, fight (run, hide, fight).

This does not mean you must physically engage with the threat. But it does mean you must take immediate, intentional action. What action to take depends on the type of threat. The FBI suggests the following sequence of actions: run, hide, fight. Think back to the chapter on proxemics. Increasing the distance between you and attackers reduces their ability to harm you. Putting up barriers that block line of sight and interrupt projectiles makes it harder for threats to harm you. Running and hiding may not always be possible, so always understand that when confronted with a threat, your only option may be a direct physical response.

If no, proceed to the next decision point.

Does the anomaly represent a potential threat?

If yes, flight (alarm, alert, leave).

Here you've decided an anomaly is significant enough to become a potential threat, and you must act on that decision. You can raise the alarm if it is safe to do so (such as with a fire). You may alert on-site authorities, such as police officers or security guards, if appropriate. Often, the best course of action is to remove yourself and those you are responsible for from the environment where the threat exists.

If no, proceed to the next decision point.

Is the anomaly relevant?

If yes, focus (observe, interact, disrupt).

If the anomaly does not trigger a need to take action but cannot yet be dismissed, continue to focus on it. If the anomaly's cluster of cues grows, work your way back up the decision tree. If the anomaly persists and the context does not change, you may choose to engage with the anomaly if you feel safe doing so, to determine context and relevance. Another option is to create an anomaly yourself, disrupting the environment in some way to change the context and reobserve the source of your initial anomaly (something as simple as ringing the bell on a counter when no one is there).

If the anomaly is not relevant, you can dismiss it and return to observing the environment as a whole for baseline and anomalies.

Having a decision tree on hand speeds up your decision-making process. And it will become more accurate and automatic over time. Your decision tree may not look like this one. Use this one as a model, but fill it in with responses and actions that apply to you and your skill level. What's important is that you have one in place. Never let more than three decision cycles accumulate before you take some kind of action. If an anomaly stands out past this point, you need to figure out why.

Rules of Threes

When under duress, your ability to process information becomes restricted. Under normal conditions, humans can process up to seven details simultaneously. In a threatening situation, this number drops to three or fewer. This is why many of the responses to duress come in sets of three.

> Tap, Rack, Bang
> The cycle of operation that occurs when a firearm fails to fire.
> Nine, One, One
> The number to dial to reach emergency services.
> Stop, Drop, Roll
> The cycle of operation to put oneself out if on fire.
> Run, Hide, Fight
> The FBI's recommended order of response to an immediate threat.
> Fight, Flight, Focus
> The "Baseline + Anomaly = Decision" decision tree.

Additional Practices to Speed up Decision-Making

Think Like a Bad Guy

If someone were going to attack you, what would that process look like, and how would it play out? Even more important, how would you respond?

In every environment you're in, put yourself in the predator's position. How does a predator move through that environment? What vulnerabilities will a predator exploit?

Look at your home environment. Stand out front and ask yourself, "How would I break into this place?"

Building File Folders

Think of each experience as a file on a specific event you can refer back to should a similar situation occur. This gives you an advantage at assessing and responding to those situations. In addition to your experiences, you can use other means to expand your file folders.

Practice Baseline + Anomaly in places you already visit. The more you observe familiar environments, the better you can recognize baseline and anomalies in similar but unfamiliar environments. Most people have a habit of lowering their guard the closer they get to home, since the surroundings become more familiar. This is a missed opportunity. The more familiar the surroundings, the easier it is to spot an anomaly.

Use other people's examples. I provide some examples of my experiences and failures with situational awareness in this book. Add those to your file folders. Do the same with other credible sources. Talk to people about their experiences. Make sure to get details. Use those to expand your file folder for those types of situations.

Use visualization and imagination to walk through situations and apply your decision tree.

Three Questions to Help You Survive the Unknown

When you are in an unfamiliar place or a situation within which you have no context, experience, or file folder to draw from, start with the three situational awareness questions:

1. What is going on here?
2. What would cause someone to stand out and why?
3. What would I do about it?

Here's a quick example. You go out for a meal at a local restaurant. You grab a seat, but there's a loud guy at the bar. For the moment, it's fine. He's just had a little too much to drink. As you wait for your food, the loud guy is getting louder with each passing second. He's swearing more, and he's also getting in people's faces. His tone has shifted, too. He sounds angry. People ignore him, which makes him angrier. So he does the only thing he knows: he gets louder still.

Your food arrives, but you don't tuck into it because you want to see how this situation will resolve. Everyone is looking at the drunk while pretending he doesn't exist. No one wants to talk to him, but they want him to shut up. It goes on because people prefer the noise to the alternative, which carries the potential for violence. Their bodies are telling them to get up and get out of the area, but they ignore that instinct and sit in an awkward atmosphere.

Humans evolved in an environment where anything that moved had the potential to kill them. Those instincts are still with us, even if we don't comprehend them. The modern world desensitizes us to our intuition.

Retrain yourself so your body doesn't shut down when you need it most. Discomfort exists to give you life-preserving information. Don't ignore it. After all, I bet you listen to it when you drive.

Learning to drive is the perfect example of situational awareness mastery. We look for signals as we drive. How close are the other cars in traffic? Is anyone speeding or cutting people off? This is a near-universal experience among adults.

Driving is the practice of situational awareness. But we often turn off that awareness when we get out of the car. Break out of that habit.

Situational awareness and the other skills covered in this book are necessary for survival. They enable you to assess risk and make the quickest decision possible. It's a lifelong habit that will serve you—and save you—in any situation.

Quick decision-making isn't just useful for threat assessment because we don't always have perfect information. In fact, we never do. And that lack of information can paralyze us until it's too late to act. Taking the right action with imperfect information is the default state of the surviving human. Use the tools you were born with to increase your chances of survival, no matter what situation you're in.

CHAPTER 15

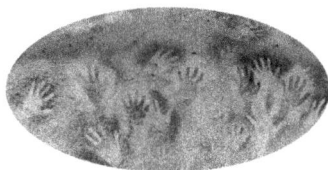

FEAR FACTOR: HARNESSING THE ESSENTIAL NEGATIVE EMOTION

What's your earliest memory? Was it a happy one? Being held by your mother? Receiving a favorite childhood toy as a gift? Lucky you . . . mine is one of fear. It was so pure to my young brain that it has been seared in there with such crystal clarity that I can still see it to this day.

When I was three years old, I was having a nightmare. In this dream, I was running through a forest from a hulking beast. My little legs stumbled, and I fell. All I could see were shadows and teeth.

Right before the monster struck, I woke up. My bed was drenched with what I hoped was sweat. In the corner of my room, I saw the outline of a figure. Had the creature followed me out of the dream world?

In that moment, I was more afraid than I'd ever been before. I wanted to scream for my mother, but when I opened my mouth, no sound came out. That memory has stuck with me over the years. It introduced me to undiluted fear and served as a demonstration of the body's automatic fear response.

What still fascinates me about that incident is that even though I was three years old, my body knew better than my brain. It would not let me make a sound.

Look at it from an ancient perspective. If the shadow beast had been real, making a sound would have alerted it to my location. That's why being so terrified you can't make a sound is a defense mechanism.

Our bodies know what to do in life-or-death situations, real or imagined. Our cognitive processes can get in the way of our bodies' innate wisdom.

When a ball, a fist, or a custard pie comes at your face, you draw back. Flinching is an immediate, innate response. These instincts have kept human beings alive. The problem is that now we think we're too good for it. We have a tendency to dismiss our innate responses in favor of logic and analysis.

That is a big mistake. Here's why.

Your Relationship with Fear

I have had a great many troubles, but most of them never happened.

—Mark Twain

There is no nice way to put this. The institutions of authority tell you that everyone is the same, and you must dismiss differences in appearance and behavior. And those institutions are lying to you. Condescending do-gooders who tell you to ignore nonverbal communication are also lying to you. The media-industrial complex manipulates your evolved abilities with loaded language and images to put you into a constant state of anxious agitation.

Your parents might be good people, but they're still lying to you. They might be pleasant lies, like "Santa Claus is coming to town," but they're lies, nonetheless. In fact, parents and most other adults are lying to kids. Many lie through omission. If you "do the right thing and be the better person," they say, nothing bad will ever happen to you.

You've never been taught about the real dangers that exist. Or how to read and understand the language of violence. If you'd been taught, you would not be reading this book.

Even you are lying to yourself. Your mind loves to overestimate your abilities. And the barman in your brain will mix up a hormonal cocktail of dopamine, endorphins, and oxytocin. It'll make you feel invincible.

Instead, get the barman to reach down for the special bottle and pour you a straight shot of cortisol. Then you'll feel the most primal of emotions: fear.

Fear is a signal that will trigger your autonomic decision-making process. It goes by a more simple name: intuition.

Intuition is a compilation of all the environmental anomalies your conscious mind ignores that will trigger an appropriate response at the subconscious level. A fear signal will stimulate immediate action in response to any perceived threat with the potential to cause pain or death.

The lies you're told, the lies you allow yourself to believe undermine your fear signal. Those lies dull your intuition. They instruct you to ignore what your limbic system tells you.

Ignoring the limbic system is a risk. It may be alerting you to an active threat nearby. Even your imagination running wild with possibilities can distract you from real signals. Over time, the lies weaken your ability to recognize the signal until it's too late.

Don't get me wrong, I get the appeal of the lie. In the lie, there is peace and love for all mankind and animals alike. The lie is easy. But it will get you killed.

The truth, on the other hand, will keep you alive.

Signal versus Emotion

You've been told that fear is an emotion, like anger and happiness. In the sense that emotions are direct, immediate feedback responses to our surroundings, that's correct.

But most people don't use the term *fear* to describe the active signal. I prefer to use *dread*, which is not an active fear signal but the anticipation of that signal. It's the feeling of waiting for fear to show up.

The Fear Scale

When we panic, we're being overwhelmed by fear signals. It means we failed to respond to previous stages of the fear scale. This scale, in descending order, is as follows:

Dread → Fright → Anxiety → Apprehension → Worry → Doubt → Concern

All these mental states are associated with fear, but they're not responses to fear. The only proper response to fear is to take action.

When we allow ourselves to sit in anticipation of fear, we make it more difficult to recognize and respond to fear signals. It begins with a feeling of doubt. Then doubt can trigger hesitation. Sustained hesitation leaves us feeling anxious about what may happen until something happens or does not. And if it does happen, that anxiety can manifest itself further and leave you in a state of panic.

Panic is not productive fear. And speaking of what fear is not . . .

What FEAR Really Is

Perhaps you've come across the following acronyms:

FEAR
False evidence appearing real

FEAR
False expectations appearing real

Both are accurate, but if you cling too tightly to those definitions, you run the risk of undermining your ability to receive the fear signal. *False* does not always mean *wrong*. It can simply mean "not right at this moment."

While it is important to recognize false alarms, you should not dismiss the potential for danger. Instead, add it to your calm assessment of the situation, and shift back to being open to signals from your environment.

Not All the Same

Throughout this book, you have had frequent exposure to the concept of anomalies. Anything that encourages you to ignore deviations in norms, dress, behavior, proximity, et cetera is working against your ability to recognize anomalies.

When you are encouraged to ignore anomalies, understand that it comes at a cost. In most cases, you are trading your awareness of the environment for comfort.

So why would anyone discourage situational awareness?

Captured Attention

There's money to be made in keeping you afraid. Many industries recognize how powerful fear is. If they can leverage that fear signal, they claim its power.

Think of how popular horror movies are. From *Nosferatu* to *The Texas Chainsaw Massacre*, horror has always brought in profits. Only one industry does it better: the mainstream news.

The news takes great care in crafting language designed to trigger conscious associations with your fear signals. They are deliberate in their use of provocative images that take advantage of those same associations. The longer they can keep you watching them to find out what is happening and what happens next (instead of relying on your own developed skills), the better it is for their bottom line.

But the news has no end. There is no final bulletin. The story goes on forever. There is always some new fear lurking round the corner ready to jump out at you. In fact, their entire business model is predicated on endless fear.

This constant barrage of false signals interferes with genuine fear signals. One of the most ingenious aspects of the news is it leaves you feeling helpless. You cannot take action on the majority of what you see on the news. All you can do is keep watching, which leaves you in a perpetual state of anxiety. That's bad news for you, but good news for the advertisers.

As we discussed, constant anxiety with no outlet can lead to panic. And panicking people make poor decisions.

The underlying mainstream narrative fosters low-grade panic. (Pay attention to how many advertisers are pharmaceutical companies selling antianxiety drugs.)

And that's just newscasters with a profit motive. The damage they can do pales in comparison to ideologues putting their thumbs on the scales to manipulate you.

When I was serving, I would get twenty-four-hour shifts. During those long shifts, the TVs would be on. And they would always be tuned to some news station. Without wanting to, I would find myself watching the news.

I soon realized that not much news happens in twenty-four hours. The news channels would milk the same story over again and again. They would cut from the anchor at the desk to someone out in the field. Then they'd bring on their analyst, then another analyst to analyze the first analyst, ad infinitum.

Forget turtles; it's analysts all the way down.

Newscasters had much more credibility back when they only had thirty minutes to read the news. Now the news industry is beholden to advertisers. It's sad that their business depends on keeping you stressed out, hopeless, and in a constant state of dread.

Because your fear should be saved for the real, direct, and immediate threats out there.

The World Is Not a Safe Place

By default, man is naked, alone, and destitute. And the entire universe is trying to kill him.

Do not be fooled. You're not safe anywhere. The illusion of safety is a comforting lie you tell yourself to justify surrendering responsibility. But understand that no matter what, you are always responsible for your situational awareness and being able to address immediate threats.

Think about it for a moment. Every day, we are surrounded by dangerous machines moving at lethal speeds. And these machines are operated by the deadliest creature to ever walk the earth. Safety is an illusion.

Yet we can and do navigate those dangers safely.

We evolved to do just that. Our senses work together to gather signals about our surroundings. The limbic system uses those signals to trigger immediate responses to keep us safe.

All the effort you put into making your surroundings safer is valuable. But nothing has more impact than developing your situational awareness and keeping yourself in a state of relaxed readiness. You are the first responder to anything that threatens your safety.

One of the hardest lessons to learn on managing fear is imagining the worst thing you can do to another person. If you can conjure it up, you have it within you to do it.

All evil done in the world is done by people. People with the same needs you and I have. When people's needs go unmet, there is physiological dysregulation we can pick up on.

This is not advanced navy SEAL training. Even infants can tell the difference between mother (food, affection) and father (play).

Those willing to commit acts of evil know, to some extent, that they must hide their intent. Some are better at hiding it than others. To paraphrase the Bible, some will appear as angels of light.

Trying too hard is also a signal. This is why "stranger danger" is still a colloquialism. An unknown person who approaches you is a threat, and kids know that. The stereotype of child sexual predators luring children with toys and candy exists for a reason. Someone who seems too good to be true usually is and should not be trusted.

Scammers who prey on the finances, health, and safety of adults use a similar tactic. The problem is we have been desensitized to forget what we knew as children. So we fall for the ploy hook, line, and sinker.

The world is not a safe place, but we can navigate it safely. Recognize the danger, and plot your route accordingly. There are efforts from all sides to deprogram this instinct. "Everything is good," we're told. "You are invincible and will live forever."

As nice as it sounds, do not listen to that narrative. Remember to always be assessing your situation.

And know how to act in the presence of fear.

The Opposite of Fear?

It is a common mistake to see fear as the opposite of courage. It's not. Courage only exists in the presence of fear. Discouragement is the opposite of courage. Emotional collapse, psychological collapse, demoralization, anger, resentment, resignation, and depression are the marks of the discouraged.

Those systems and institutions that benefit from your dependence want you demoralized and discouraged. That way, you can only navigate your fear through them.

The term *oppression* pops up a lot these days. Not to downplay it, but *discouragement* is more accurate when it comes to describing what people are feeling now. They are being denied the means to navigate their fear.

Another overused word—*privilege*—is applied to people who navigate their fear successfully. The observer sees the "privileged" act in their own interest despite their fears and assumes that is only possible because the privileged have no reason to fear. The observer can't figure out how the privileged are able to act the way they do. That assumes the privileged must have some kind of outside benefit the observer does not receive.

Look at it like this: the privileged acts in spite of fear; the observer acts *because of* fear.

Improving your competence using the lessons in this book will free you from helpless dependence on others for basic survival. Replacing helplessness and dread with competence and confidence will reverse your dependent behavior and restore strategies of self-determination.

Fear will either blunt you into helplessness or sharpen you into competence. Act accordingly.

CHAPTER 16

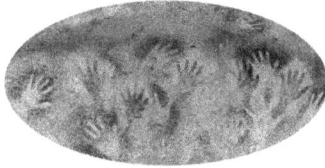

WE'RE ALL MICE NOW: CORE HUMAN COMPETENCE IN OUR POSTMODERN DYSTOPIA

How are you like a mouse? Before you shout that you're lactose intolerant, this has nothing to do with any cheese aversion you might have.

Let me introduce you to Professor John B. Calhoun. In the 1970s, he ran a series of experiments that investigated what would happen if mice had all their needs catered to. Professor Calhoun came up with the mouse utopia. The most famous of these utopias was Universe 25.

Calhoun took four pairs of eight mice: sixteen males and sixteen females. The mice had unlimited food and water, the temperature was kept at a mouse-perfect 68° F, and bedding was furnished.

With food and shelter provided and a lot of free time on their paws, you can guess what happened next. That's right. They filled their time with squeaky mouse sex. There was a population explosion. Every 55 days, the population doubled. It continued to increase until it got to 620, when growth slowed. After that, Universe 25's mouse count would only double every 145 days.

The mouse populace split into groups. Those that could not find a group became isolated.

Can you see where I'm going with this?

Let's continue. It'll become apparent soon.

The males who could not fit in withdrew physically and psychologically. Their movement dropped to almost zero, and they congregated in the foyer area of Universe 25. They ceased all interaction with their fellow mice. In fact, they were such nonentities that even the most territorial male mice wouldn't bother to attack them. That doesn't mean they came out unscathed. They were attacked by other withdrawn males that got too close. Some of the withdrawn males wouldn't even defend themselves.

There were female mice with no place, too. Instead of whipsawing between bouts of lethargy and extreme violence like their male counterparts, they focused on themselves. They would spend days preening and grooming themselves. These females became so vain, they would shun mating altogether. Calhoun referred to these mice as the "beautiful ones."

Odd behavior wasn't limited to the outsiders. In-group behavior was altered, too. Alpha male mice had heightened aggression. They would attack others for no reason. The alphas would rape both males and females, and the more violent encounters would end in acts of cannibalism.

Mommy mice would abandon their young or forget about them, leaving the newborns to fend for themselves. Mothers also directed aggression at males, sometimes the fathers of their brood. These deadbeat dads would be exiled to join the outsiders.

The moms' violence was even directed at the children. Mothers would kill their young. In some sections of Universe 25, infant mortality was 90 percent.

It didn't end there. Calhoun termed the first phase "Mouse 1984." The next phase had the optimistic title "Second Death." That phase concerned the mice that survived the violent moms. They grew up exhibiting strange behaviors. Because their mothers had been psychotic, they never learned how to act like mice. In a permanent state of arrested development, they showed no interest in mating. Instead, they groomed and ate all day.

Universe 25's population peaked at 2,200, even though it could have held up to 3,000. Many of the Second Death–generation mice retired to their own areas. Others grouped into violent gangs that would cannibalize other groups of mice and those in their own group, too.

With all the violence, low birth rate, and high infant mortality, the population cratered. The fate of the remaining mice was sealed. It's important to note that at no point did food, water, or shelter ever run out.

Calhoun coined the term *behavioral sink* to explain the collapse. He wrote in the conclusion to his study "For an animal so simple as a mouse, the most complex behaviors involve the interrelated set of courtship, maternal care, territorial defense, and hierarchical intragroup and inter-group social organization."

Humans are more complex than rodents, but not by much. If you learn nothing else, know that even if you live in the land of plenty, things can always go south. Even having food, water, and shelter doesn't excuse letting yourself become complacent.

And a major cause of complacency is modern convenience. With the best of intentions, we've created our own utopia of comfort and convenience, and we have become the mice.

The Convenience Regression

We've gone from being tool-making apex predators to blowing ourselves up by reheating a day-old burrito in the microwave. We evolved to hunt and gather, but we've traded the risks of self-determination for the ease and comfort of dependence. Now we're completely reliant on others to meet our core needs.

You are a hostage to the supply chain.

When humans abandon our adaptive generalist foundation, we make a rapid descent down the links in the food chain. Our adaptability, though still just as efficient, gets blunted by an overreliance on comfort. Every convenience we've leveraged comes to replace our competence, and instead of being a platform to lift us higher, it becomes a crutch.

We delude ourselves by calling our dependencies "conveniences." Many outright deny how much self-determination we've traded for comfort. The conveniences cover our access to:

- Food
- Water
- Shelter
- Safety
- Security

It's not enough for these needs to be met. Doing that will make you dependent. You'll become anxious to keep your providers amenable so they'll continue to provide for you. In order to rise above dependence and become a fully developed human, able to sustain your own survival, you must develop the basic skill to provide for yourself. Your limbic system knows the difference.

And providing for yourself depends on navigating human interaction.

Three Categories of Human Interaction to Remember: Cooperation, Avoidance (Boycott), and Violence

Cooperation is a voluntary exchange of commensurate value—interactions that produce benefits. Avoidance is the choice not to engage—interactions that produce neither benefits nor harms. Violence is the application or threat of force—interactions that produce harm.

Much of what people consider cooperation today is, instead, violence. They are responding to a compulsion, not acting voluntarily. "It's easier if I just go along" is not cooperation; it's closer to coercion.

My goal is to keep the opportunity for cooperation alive. We cannot cooperate when we are incompetent. Building competence for sustaining life is the foundation of every other vector of human interaction. In an ideal world, we aim to cooperate. But our ability to cooperate is restricted by our competence. Dependence is not cooperation.

How We're Compromising Ourselves Every Day

When you rely on others to keep you alive, it's crucial that you don't do anything to piss them off. If you get cast out, what will you do? Being dependent on others can be detrimental to your health.

People don't comprehend the extent to which we have become dependent on systems. Yet these systems couldn't care less if we died. Worst of all, they exist only because so many are convinced they're essential for survival. But we don't need what these systems teach us we require. Wants and preferences are being sold as requirements.

These systems don't teach you what you do need. Think of everything you depend on just to meet your basic needs. Each of these is a lever of compulsion that can be used to control you. There are food levers, water levers, shelter levers, and even violence levers.

My goal in writing this book is to empower people to say no and mean it. The more ways we can counter, find alternatives, or outright refuse to participate, the weaker today's systems of control become.

The Cooperation Problem

Healthy societies layer divisions of labor and specializations on a foundation of skills and practices that secure self-determination. This ensures these efforts remain valuable forms of cooperation rather than dependencies that become vulnerabilities.

But our society is not healthy.

We have overcommitted to our division of labor. Instead of layering specialization on a core set of human competencies, we layer specialization on dependencies.

Specialization must be layered on generalization, never replace it.

And these skills must be handed down from one generation to the next.

Forever Young?

But we no longer pass on life-sustaining skills to the next generation. We have been manipulated into coddling the insecure. And the immature behavior expected of children is now tolerated in adults.

Our society suffers from pathological neoteny, extending childhood behavioral flexibility well into neurological maturity. This societal disorder is characterized by the extension of childish trappings into adulthood. Symptoms include:

- Suspended maturation
- Suppressed development
- Inappropriate dependence
- Unregulated emotion
- Misplaced attention

Somewhere along the way, we started treating adults like children. We managed our expectations, but some of us were shocked whenever we encountered adults behaving like kids. They didn't even behave like good kids. Instead, they behaved like spoiled brats.

This may come as a shock, but adults behaving like kids is not good. In fact, we won't solve any other social problem until we restore adult self-determination. If you make room in the playpen for children and adults, the kids will be the ones who lose out. Remember Calhoun's Second Death phase?

Systems of control benefit from our dependence. They want childhood extended until the line between child and adult disappears. This instills learned helplessness and lets them push childlike make-believe as reality. So it's no surprise when what used to be a phase people went through becomes a permanent identity.

This sustained childhood has even been institutionalized. US insurance law allows children to be on their parents' insurance as dependents until they are twenty-six years old.

Everything in this book is remedial adulthood. I saw that phenomenon, and I wanted to go as far back as I could to address it.

That's where survival skills come into play. Humans are unique in our default unpreparedness for the wilderness but also in our ability to learn to survive.

The "woke" phenomenon is the mental frame of a person under low pressure to mature. The woke have a childlike, self-centered concept of reality: not in some abstract way, but at the level of cognition. They represent a failure to mature and develop.

Nature doesn't subsidize dysfunction; it punishes suboptimal strategies. Like the private sector, it expects results. The rest of civilization is sliding toward the cliff edge, but you can walk away. If you are a parent or teacher, impart these lessons to the children in your care. Do not do to this generation what the previous one did to you.

What does it look like to integrate these skills into everyday life? It's going on a hike with your friends and pointing out and consuming the edible plants you find. It's teaching buddies how to find and prepare drinking water when you go camping. And it's being aware of everyone within twenty-five feet at all times. Your gut instinct talks; you listen.

These skills separate humans from animals. With them, a capable adult human can survive.

Cooperation requires you to have the ability to refuse. To be able to choose not to cooperate. Otherwise, there is no choice, and what you are doing is something other than cooperating. The foundational human core competencies developed in this book give you the option of avoidance. Situational awareness paired with the ability to sustain your own existence empower you to avoid violence and preserve the opportunity for cooperation. When the system makes any demand of you, you now have the capacity to say yes and cooperate completely of your own volition or to say no and mean it.

This book may have been your first exposure to these survival skills. Don't get me wrong. This is not bushcraft survival training. What I've taught you are human skills. They allow an adult human to survive in the environment and collaborate with others. This is the foundation of cooperation, and cooperation is what took us from drinking from streams to flushing toilets indoors. We got *here* because of who we were *there*.

Reading this book will not tell you everything you need to know. It will provide you with the absolute minimum. To integrate this knowledge into your life, gain competence in these skills, and remember them when it counts, I suggest getting the video book version of *The Primal Primer*.

Our civilization already forgot how to survive once. Let's not forget again.

To help you remember, I've created a video book companion to *The Primal Primer*. If you found yourself forgetting important lessons or takeaways or you skipped a few (or several) sections, the video book is for you. If you're a visual learner, perfect. We'll make sure the most important lessons of *The Primal Primer* stick with you for life.

Visit www.lukeweinhagen.com/videobook to get a copy of the video book. You'll get 50% off with discount code MASTERY.

Thank you for reading this book and investing in your own core human competence. Talk to me anytime on Twitter @LukeWeinhagen or email me at luke@lukeweinhagen.com.

RECOMMENDED READING

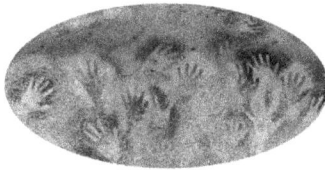

Aristotle. *On the Soul.* Translated by J.A. Smith. Cambridge, MA: MIT (The Internet Classics Archive), c. 350 BCE.

Boothman, Nicholas. *How to Make People Like You in 90 Seconds or Less.* New York: Workman Publishing Company, Inc., 2000.

Carnegie, Dale. *How to Win Friends and Influence People.* New York: Gallery Books, 1936.

De Becker, Gavin. *The Gift of Fear.* New York: Dell Publishing, 1997.

Dutton, Edward. *How to Judge People by What They Look Like.* Independently Published, 2018.

Givens, David, PhD. *Crime Signals: How to Spot a Criminal Before You Become a Victim.* New York: St. Martin's Press, 2008.

Gladwell, Malcolm. *Blink: The Power of Thinking without Thinking.* New York: Little, Brown and Company, 2005.

Kahneman, Daniel. *Thinking Fast and Slow.* New York: Farrar, Straus and Giroux, 2011.

Klein, Gary. *Sources of Power: How People Make Decisions.* Cambridge, MA: MIT Press, 1998.

Livingston, Eustace Hazard (Ed). *The Trapper's Bible: The Most Complete Guide to Trapping and Hunting Tips Ever.* New York: Skyhorse Publishing, 2012.

Maslow, A.H. "A Theory of Human Motivation." *Psychological Review* 50 (1943): 370–396.

Maslow, A.H. *The Farther Reaches of Human Nature.* New York: Viking Press, 1971.

Medina, John. *Brain Rules*: *12 Principles for Surviving and Thriving at Work, Home, and School*. Seattle: Pear Press, 2008.

Navaro, Joe, *What Every Body Is Saying: An Ex-FBI Agent's Guide to Speed-Reading People*. New York: HarperCollins Publishers, 2008.

Pease, Allan and Barbara *The Definitive Book of Body Language: The Hidden Meaning behind People's Gestures and Expressions*. New York: Bantam Dell, 2004.

Press, Gerald A. (Ed). *The Continuum Companion to Plato*. London and New York: Continuum International Publishing Group, 2012.

Rately, John J., MD, with Eric Hagerman. *Spark: The Revolutionary New Science of Exercise and the Brain*. New York: Little, Brown and Company, 2008.

Van Horn, Patrick, and Jason A. Riley. *Left of Bang: How the Marine Corps' Combat Hunter Program Can Save Your Life*. New York: Black Irish Entertainment LLC, 2014.

Vallentyne, J.R., PhD. *Tragedy in Mouse Utopia: An Ecological Commentary on Human Utopia*. Bloomington, IN: Trafford Publishing, 2006.

Voss, Chris *Never Split the Difference: Negotiating As If Your Life Depended On It*. New York: HarperCollins Publishing, 2016.

ACKNOWLEDGMENTS

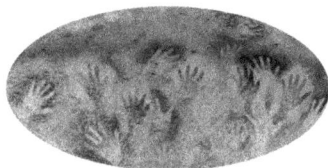

A project like this is not possible without the support of others. My thanks go to my wife, Malia, and my family for making room in our lives for me to focus on this material.

Thank you to my peers at the Natural Law Institute for shaping and sharpening the ideas that led to this writing.

Thank you to Yousef Badou and his team at Emergence Disrupt LLC for the fantastic training in situational awareness and behavioral analysis.

Thank you to everyone at the Entrepreneur's Wordsmith for providing the structure to make this project possible. I am grateful to you all.

ABOUT THE AUTHOR

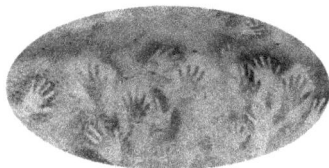

Luke Weinhagen is a certified situation awareness instructor, former United States Marine, and the creator of Dangerously Competent, a self-defense and self-sufficiency training program. For over twenty-five years, Luke has taught individuals, families, and organizations to assess risk, respond swiftly, and win. He is the author of *The Primal Primer* and a practical philosophy fellow at the Natural Law Institute. Learn more about Luke's training materials at www.lukeweinhagen.com.

www.ingramcontent.com/pod-product-compliance
Lightning Source LLC
Chambersburg PA
CBHW031432270326
41930CB00007B/677